Medicine & Society
In America

Medicine & Society
In America

Advisory Editor

Charles E. Rosenberg
Professor of History
University of Pennsylvania

CATECHISM

OF

HEALTH

FOR THE

USE OF SCHOOLS,

AND FOR

DOMESTIC INSTRUCTION.

By B. C. FAUST, M. D.

ARNO PRESS & THE NEW YORK TIMES
New York   1972

Reprint Edition 1972 by Arno Press Inc.

Reprinted from a copy in
The Library of The College of
Physicians of Philadelphia

LC# 74-180574
ISBN 0-405-03951-4

Medicine and Society in America
ISBN for complete set: 0-405-03930-1
See last pages of this volume for titles.

Manufactured in the United States of America

CATECHISM

OF

HEALTH:

FOR THE

USE OF SCHOOLS,

AND FOR

DOMESTIC INSTRUCTION.

———————

By B. C. FAUST, M. D.

Counsellor and Physician to the Reigning Count of Schaumburgh Lippe; Fellow of the Royal Society of Economy at Potsdam; of the Helvetic Corresponding Society of Physicians and Surgeons; and of the Royal Society of Agriculture at Celle, in the Electorate of Hanover.

———————

TRANSLATED FROM THE LAST IMPROVED GERMAN
EDITION OF THIS WORK,

BY J. H. BASSE.

═══════════════

DUBLIN:

PRINTED BY P. BYRNE, (108) GRAFTON-STREET.

1794.

⁎ *The* FRONTISPIECE *represents a* CHILD *in a loose Garment, such as all Children from the Beginning of the Third, to the End of the Seventh or Eighth Year, ought to wear.*

TO

SCHOOLMASTERS;

ON THE USE OF THE

CATECHISM OF HEALTH.

WORTHY and respectable Members of Society, you love those Children that are sent to you to be educated, to imbibe such Instructions and Doctrines as will render them Healthy, Sensible, Virtuous, and Happy.

This Book teaches how Man from his infancy ought to live, in order to enjoy a perfect State of Health, which, as Sirach says, is better than gold. You will, therefore, with pleasure, I hope, instruct your dear little Pupils in its principles; and as able and experienced Men, convinced that the mere learning of the Answers by heart can be of no advantage to Children, you will have no objection to instruct them after the following method.

1. The Chapter which is chosen for Instruction ought first to be read by the Master, and then by two Children that read perfectly well and distinct; one of them reading the Questions, the other the Answers regularly and in order to the end of the Chapter; the Master, understanding thoroughly what has been read, explains its general import.

2. He then explains each Query and Answer particularly, and the meaning of the words and ideas. He elucidates Answers and resolves Questions, consisting sometimes of more than one Sentence, in a concise, simple manner, easily conceivable by the intellects of Children. He converses with them, and, in a perspicuous manner, by easy, simple, and slowly progressive Questions, inculcates the Truths and Doctrines contained in the Chapter.

The Queries and Answers ought to follow each other in regular and natural order, that the Children by their own judgment and understanding may find out and conceive what is true and good.

After they are perfectly acquainted with the true meaning of one Query and Answer, the next is introduced, and so on, till they are made familiar with the true intent and meaning of them all singly.

3. The Master then examines the Children through the whole Chapter. If he finds that they are well acquainted with its contents, the Lecture is concluded by repeating what has been taught,

taught, and by asking each child "What he or she remembers of it?"

4. The Master then asks the following Questions, leading to Answers different from those already given:—

"Which of you would now, after those salutary instructions, do such or such mischief?"— "Would not you do such a thing, so or so?"— "Would not you repeat such or such a thing to your parents or friends at home?"—"How would you contrive it, that such or such a custom might be altered, or things done in such a way, as, from what you heard just now, they ought to be done?"—"Do you know any body whom you could benefit by acquainting him with what you have learned to-day?"—"Which of those excellent rules for your future conduct have you resolved to follow?"

5. The subjoined Observations will enable a Master possessed of any judgment to explain and confirm many truths, that will be both instructive and pleasing to his Pupils.

6. When, for instance, a Fever, Small-pox, Measles, Flux, or other Disease, rages in the neighbourhood, the Chapter that treats of those maladies ought to be frequently, and in preference of all others, read.

7. An hour, at least, twice a week, ought to be devoted to such Instruction, in order that the whole CATECHISM of HEALTH may be gone through twice a year, and the minds of the

Children

Children impressed with the true spirit of its doctrine.

In this manner, my worthy friends, I beseech you to instruct your pupils; and if you do so, rest assured, that the present, as well as future generations will be under obligations to you for their Health and Happiness; and the Almighty whose Divine Will it is that all Mankind should be rendered temporally and eternally happy through the knowledge of truth, and who leaves nothing unrewarded, will reward you according to your different degrees of Merit, in this and in the World to come.

FIRST DIVISION.

OF HEALTH.

I. *Of Health; its Value, and the Duty of preserving it, and of instructing Mankind, particularly Children, in these important Subjects.*

Q. 1. DEAR Children, to breathe, to live in this world, created by God, is it an advantage? is it to enjoy happiness and pleasure?

A. Yes. To live is to enjoy happiness and pleasure; for life is a precious gift of the Almighty.

Ps. cl. 6. Let every thing that has breath praise the Lord.

Ps. cxlv. 16. Thou, O Lord, satisfiest the desire of every thing living.

Ps. xxxvi. 5, 8. Thy mercy, O Lord, is in the heavens; and thy faithfulness reacheth unto the clouds. They shall be abundantly satisfied with the fatness of thy house; and thou shalt make them drink of the river of thy pleasures.

Ps. cxxxvi. 1, 8, 9, 25. O give thanks unto the Lord, for he is good. To him that made the sun, to rule by the day; the moon and stars to rule by night; who gives food to all flesh: for his mercy endureth for ever.

Q. 2. What other proofs have we to shew that life is an excellent gift of God?

A. The instinct, or natural anxiety of mankind to preserve it.

Q. 3. What must be the state of the human body the habitation and slave of the soul, that man may enjoy a long, prosperous and happy life?

A. It

A. It muft be healthy.

Q. 4. How elfe can you prove that man ought to be in a good ftate of health?

A. By the commandment of God, *viz.* " In the " fweat of thy face fhalt thou eat bread." Gen. iii. 19.

Q. 5. Can we poffibly promote the perfection and happinefs of our fouls, if we do not take proper care of our bodies?

A. No. God has fo intimately united foul and body, that by a rational care taken of the body the happinefs and purity of the foul is increafed.

Q. 6. What is underftood by a ftate of good health?

A. That the body is free from pains and infirmities, fulfils its duties cheerfully and with eafe, and is always obedient to the foul.

Q. 7. How does he feel who enjoys health?

A. Strong; full of vigour and power; he relifhes his meals; is not affected by wind and weather; goes through exercife and labour with eafe, and feels himfelf always happy.

Q. 8. And what are the fenfations of the fick? Are they like thofe we have defcribed?

A. By no means; the fick man feels himfelf weak and feeble; he has no appetite; he cannot work, nor brave wind and weather; he labours under continual anxiety and pains, and very few are the pleafures of his life.

Q. 9. Can you children be merry and laugh, joke, and jump about, eat, drink and fleep, when you are ill?

A. No. We can only do fo when we are in good health.

OBSERVATION.

If a child be prefent who was ill not long ago, the Mafter will take the opportunity of afking him the following queftion:——" You was ill; tell me, did you feel yourfelf fo happy, fo eafy, as you do now?" To this a fenfible child will anfwer, swer, or will be taught to answer—" I found myself exceedingly ill, I could neither eat, drink, nor sleep; nothing afforded me pleasure or joy; I was full of anxiety and pains; but now restored to health, thanks be to God, I know it is the greatest good."

Q. 10. The blessings of health then must be very great?

A. They are indeed. Health is the most precious good, and the most certain means of enjoying all other blessings and pleasures of life.

Q. 11. What says Sirach of health?

A. In the 30th Chapter, v. 14, 15, 16, he says, " Better is the poor being found and strong of constitution, than a rich man that is afflicted in his body. Health and good estate of body are above all gold, and a strong body above infinite wealth. There is no riches above a sound body, and no joy above the joy of the heart.

Q. 12. Cannot the sick as well as the healthy, enjoy the blessings and pleasures of life?

A. No. They have no charms for the sick.

Q. 13. Of what use then is all worldly happiness to him who is sick, and cannot enjoy it?

A. Of very little use, if any.

Q. 14. If then health be the most precious boon of life, what duties has a man in that respect to discharge towards himself?

A. He must strive to preserve it.

Q. 15. Is it sufficient if he take care of his own health?

A. No. It is also his duty to take care of the life and health of his fellow-creatures.

Q. 16. And what is the duty of parents toward their children?

A. They are bound to take the tenderest care of their health and life.

OBSERVATION.

School-masters and parents ought to seize every opportunity of impressing on the minds of their children,

children, the great importance of the invaluable blessings of health, and the consequent duty to preserve it, by innocent pleasures, conducive to a great accession of health. They ought, on the other hand, to point out the mournful instances of multiplied sorrows and miseries which present themselves daily to our view, in the persons of the sick and diseased.

Q. 17. Do they fulfil this duty?
A. Very seldom.
Q. 18. Why so seldom?
A. 1. Because few of them are sensible of the real value of health.

2. Most of them are ignorant of the structure and state of the human body.

3. Equally ignorant of what is conducive or hurtful to health.

Q. 19. What is the cause of this ignorance?
A. The want of proper instructions.

Q. 20. But as God wills the happiness of all mankind, should they not be brought from ignorance to the knowledge of truth?

A. Yes. It would be right, good, and dutiful to instruct every body, particularly little children like us, and to teach us the structure of the human body, and the best means of preserving health.

Q. 21. Is it not, therefore, your duty to pay the greatest attention to the instructions which you are now to receive, respecting the most valuable boon of life?

A. We shall exert ourselves to the utmost to understand and to remember them.

Q. 22. Is it sufficient to receive those instructions, and to remember them?

A. No. We should also strictly conform ourselves to those instructions.

OBSERVATION.

At the close of 1791, when many, through ignorance, fell victims to the baneful influence of the

the bloody-flux, the Dowager Princefs Juliana of Schaumburgh Lippe, firft conceived the bleffed idea of caufing a Catechifm of Health to be written and publifhed for the ufe of Schools, and inftruction of children.

This Catechifm, in an imperfect ftate, appeared in 1792, yet eighty thoufand copies of it were fold, and it was introduced into fchools as a book of inftruction.

II. *Of the Duration of Life, and the Signs of Health.*

Q. 23. WHAT is the ufual period of human life?

A. Life is the beft gift of God to man, who ought to enjoy it a very long time, and therefore live to an old age, as was intended.

Pf. lxxxx. 10. The days of our life are threefcore years and ten, and if by reafon of ftrength they be fourfcore years.

OBSERVATION.

According to the ftructure of the human body, the long bones of the limbs confift till the eighteenth year of three pieces, that they may grow after that time longitudinally till the period of adult age; and this wife difpofition in the ftructure of the body would be without defign, if man were deftined to die in his infancy. Befide, from the whole nature of man, it can be proved, that he is formed to live a long time, till body and foul have attained their ultimate degree of perfection; till the body is wore out, and the foul has accomplifhed its deftination, then the one is to return into the bofom of nature, and the other into the hands of the Almighty, there to remain till the happy day of eternal blifs The tears of parents on the mournful occafion of the early demife of their infants, are therefore very juft.

Q. 24.

Q. 24. What has God promised as the greatest earthly reward to those that honour father and mother, and keep his commandments?

A. That their days shall be long upon the land, which the Lord our God gives them.

Q. 25. How long is man destined to enjoy health?

A. He ought to live almost uninterruptedly in a perfect state of health.

Q. 26. What epithet is applied to a man who only, at intervals, suffers little inconveniencies from a short illness?

A. The epithet *healthy*.

Q. 27. What epithet is applied to a man who is, not only weak, but also spends the greatest part of his life on the bed of sickness?

A The epithet *unhealthy*.

Q. 28. What are the signs of an uninterrupted state of health, enjoyed by a man at the age of maturity?

A. The fresh and healthy colour of his face, the quickness of his senses, the strength of his bones, and the firmness of his flesh; large veins full of blood; a large and full breast; the power of breathing slowly and deep without coughing; eating with hunger, and digesting well; taking much exercise, and bearing continued labour without fatigue; sleeping quietly and soundly, and enjoying cheerfulness of mind and serenity of countenance; all denote an uninterrupted state of health.

OBSERVATION.

All aliment ought to consist of solid substances, adapted to the number and strength of the teeth; the teeth serve chiefly for mastication, digestion, and, of course, the nourishment, health, strength, and happiness of a man depends, in a great degree, on the mastication of the solid part of the food, which is mixed with the saliva, and converted into a sweet milk-like fluid, called chyle: it is, therefore, necessary that a healthy man should have a sound set of teeth.

Q. 29. Can

Q. 29. Can one always and solely depend upon these signs of health?

A. No. They are apt to deceive sometimes.

Q. 30. What must be done, in order, unerringly, to ascertain whether an apparently healthy man be so in reality?

A. The temperament, health, and virtuous or moral conduct of his parents, ought to be considered.

Q. 31. What ought to be the state of health of the parents of a healthy person?

A. The father as well as the mother ought to be strong and vigorous, not deformed, nor subject to such diseases as may descend to their children, *viz.* Consumption, Epilepsy, *&c.* They both ought to have a good constitution, and the prospect of attaining old age in good health, and should be of a virtuous disposition.

Q. 32. Why is it necessary for them to be virtuous?

A. Because the virtue of the parents are discovered in the children, and because virtuous parents encourage their children, by their example, to endeavour to become worthy and honourable members of society.

Q. 33. What then must be the disposition of those parents, who wish to bring up virtuous and healthy children?

A. They must be virtuous and healthy themselves.

III. *Of the Construction, or Structure, of the Human Body.*

Q. 34. How is the human body constructed?
A. With infinite wisdom and goodness, and in the most appropriate and perfect manner.

OBSERVATION.

A book of instruction for schools, on the admirable construction of the human body, and on the functions

functions of its different parts, elucidated by correct prints, ought to be, and soon will be published, being as necessary as useful.

Q. 35. What have we in particular to observe with respect to the perfect structure of the human body?

A. That it is endowed with the greatest and most appropriate powers, tending to preserve life and health, to remove diseases, or to heal wounds.

Q. 36. If the body contain any thing unnatural, or if it has been wounded, or otherwise hurt, so as to cause its functions to be obstructed, how do those powers act?

A. They operate more or less powerfully to expel from the body all that is unnatural, or to heal its wounds.

OBSERVATION.

If a splinter sticks in any part of the body, irritated nature produces matter to expel it. If the stomach be loaded with bile, or putrid matter, nature strives to remove it by vomiting. If a particular sickly state of body should become dangerous to life, nature arouses all her energy to remove it; a shivering or heat, or a fever, will generally take place, by which nature attempts to concoct the offending matter, or, what commonly happens, expel it from the body. If a person has broken one of his limbs, nature will soften the broken ends of the bone, in order that they may knit without plaister or salve: but the previous assistance of an able surgeon is required to bring the broken ends of the bone in contact, and to secure them so, after which tranquillity and rest are necessary.

Q. 37. Can the body, notwithstanding all those great powers with which God has endowed man, sustain any injury?

A. The healthy and vigorous man is very seldom subject to any.

Q. 38. But as we, neverthelefs, fee fo many objects of pity, what may be the real reafon of their fufferings?

A. Weaknefs; or the want of pure vital faculties.

Q. 39. Is this weaknefs natural?

A. No. Naturally man is ftrong, full of vigour and health.

Q. 40. How have fo many contracted this weaknefs?

A. Generally through their own faults, or through ignorance.

Q. 41. Is there not another particular reafon why men are fo weak?

A. Yes. Their weaknefs has been hereditary, and tranfmitted to them from generation to generation.

Q. 42. What muft men do, that they may be lefs expofed to ficknefs?

A. They muft do every thing to recover their natural ftrength.

OBSERVATION.

By this ftrength, you muft not underftand a rude but a cultivated ftrength, when the body is accuftomed to exercife, and is full of life and vigour.

Q. 43. By what means can man recover his natural ftrength?

A. By receiving a judicious and liberal education, and leading a prudent life.

Q. 44. By what particular means can a ftrong and healthy body be injured, or rendered unwholefome?

A. By a bad education and corrupt way of living; by intemperance in eating and drinking; by unwholefome food and fpirituous liquors; by breathing bad or unwholefome air; by uncleanlinefs; by too great exercife or inactivity; by heats and colds; by affliction, forrow, grief, and mifery; and by many other means, the human body may be injured, and loaded with difeafe.

IV. *On the Attending and Nursing of Infants.*

Q. 45. WHAT does the little helpless infant stand most in need of?

A. The love and care of his mother.

Q. 46. Can this love and care be shewn by other persons?

A. No. Nothing equals maternal love.

Q. 47. Why does a child stand so much in need of the love and care of his mother?

A. Because the attendance and nursing, the tender and affectionate treatment which a child stands in need of, can only be expected from a mother.

Q. 48. How ought infants be attended and nursed

A. They ought always to breathe fresh and pure air; be kept dry and clean, and immersed in cold water every day.

Q. 49. Why so?

A. Because children are now, at the time alluded to, more placid, because not being irritable, they grow and thrive better.

Q. 50. Is it good to swathe a child?

A. No. Swathing is a very bad custom, and produces in children great anxiety and pains; it is injurious to the growth of the body, and prevents children from being kept clean and dry.

Q. 51. Is the rocking of children proper?

A. No. It makes them uneasy, giddy, and stupid and is therefore as hurtful to the soul as to the body

Q. 52. Do children rest and sleep without being rocked?

A. Yes. If they be kept continually dry and clean, and in fresh air, they will rest and sleep well, if not disturbed; the rocking and carrying about of children is quite useless.

OBSERVATION.

As the human soul in a state of infancy is disturbed by rocking, carrying about and dancing, such practices

practices ought to be confidered as dangerous and erroneous.

The mother ought to play with the child in an affectionate and gentle manner; ought to give it frequent and bland exercife, and inftil gradually into its mind a knowledge of fuch objects as attract its notice.

Q. 53. Is it in general neceffary to keep children quiet?
A. Yes, it is.
Q. 54. What is therefore very bad?
A. The making a great noife about children; and it is ftill worfe to frighten them.
Q. 55. It is, therefore, not advifable, I fuppofe, to frighten children into fleep?
Q. By no means; becaufe they may be thrown into convulfions, and get cramps.
Q. 56. Is it neceffary or good to give children compofing draughts, or other medicines that tend to promote fleep?
A. No. They caufe an unnatural, and, of courfe, unwholefome, fleep; and are very dangerous and hurtful.
Q. 57. How long muft a mother fuckle her child?
A. For nine or twelve months.

OBSERVATION.

In fact the child ought to be fuckled till it has two teeth in each jaw. Some children are fuckled for two or three years; a practice not only erroneous, but hurtful both to mother and child.

Q. 58. What fort of aliment is prejudicial to the health of children?
A. Meal-pap, pancakes, and tough, heavy, and fat meats.
Q. 59. What harm do they do?
A. They obftruct the bowels; and childrens' bellies get, by thofe indigeftible meals, hard and fwelled.
Q. 60. What food is moft fuitable for children?
A. Pure, unadulterated new-milk, and thin gruel; grated crufts of bread; or bifcuit boiled with water only, or mixed with milk.

Q. 61. Is it proper to chew the food before you give it to children?

A. No. It is disgusting and hurtful.

OBSERVATION.

To suffer children to suck the mock-bubby, boats, &c. are very bad and disgusting customs, which occasion gripes, and therefore are dangerous.

Q. 62. What is in general to be observed with regard to the feeding of children?

A. That they be regularly and moderately fed, and their stomachs not loaded with milk or other things. It is, therefore, necessary to prevent people from giving children sweetmeats, or food out of season: the feeding of the child ought to be entirely left to its mother.

Q. 63. Do affectionate careful mothers act right when they take their infants with them to bed?

A. No. It is dangerous and hurtful; children ought, therefore, to lay by themselves.

OBSERVATION.

In Italy, mothers who take their sucklings to bed with them use the following machine, which protects them from all injury and danger. It is called *Arcuccio*, and is 3 feet 2 inches long; and the head-board 14 inches broad, and 13 inches high.

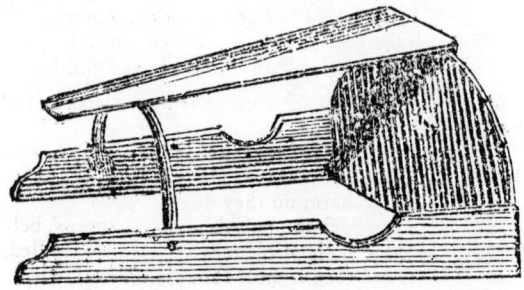

Q. 64. Is it necessary to keep infants very warm?

A. No. They must not be kept too warm.

Q. 65.

Q. 65. Is it good to cover their heads?
A. By no means; it causes humours to break out.

OBSERVATION.

From the hour of birth the head of a child ought to be kept uncovered. Mothers will find that, even in the coldest night, when they lay their hands on an infant's head, it is always warm.

Q. 66. Children are eager to stare at every thing, particularly at the light; what is to be observed with regard to this?
A. They ought to be immediately turned so as to have the object in a direct line before them; they should never be suffered to look at it sideways, as that would cause them to squint.

Q. 67. By what means is the getting of teeth rendered difficult and dangerous?
A. By caps; by keeping the head too warm; by uncleanliness and improper food.

OBSERVATION.

Nature herself causes pains at teething time, and the child is afterwards the cause of many more. It may not be amiss here to observe, 1. That pains and agonies are the first instructors of man; they teach him to avoid ills, and make him provident, compassionate, humane, and courageous. 2. Natural bodily pain, in many instances, and particularly in childhood, is less hurtful to man and his happiness, than the anxiety and mortification of soul which a child suffers that is irritated, put in a passion, or treated with contempt; and it is as bad to frighten children.

Q. 68 What is to be observed with regard to making children walk?
A. They ought not to be taught to walk in strings, or chairs, or go-carts, or be led by the arm; they ought to be suffered to creep on the floor, till by degrees they learn to walk.

Q. 69.

Q. 69. How can we best assist children in speaking?

A. We ought to pronounce the words to them very distinctly and slowly; first single sounds, and then easy words.

OBSERVATION.

It is of the greatest importance that man, from his earliest infancy, should be accustomed to a distinct pronunciation.

Q. 70. What are the principal reasons why one-fourth of the number of children that come into the world, die in the course of the first two years?

A. Want of fresh pure air, uncleanliness, bad indigestible food, particularly meal-pap; the anxiety and misery of parents are also among the causes of the death of so many children.

V. *Of the Treatment of Children with respect to their Bodies, from the Third to the Ninth or Twelfth Year.*

OBSERVATION.

FROM the third to the seventh year the child has 20 milk-teeth, and during that time the body is weak; these are changed from that period to the twelfth year for strong teeth. In the ninth year the child has 10 milk, and 12 perfect teeth. In the twelfth year both sexes have 24 strong and perfect teeth, and not until then the body begins to receive its natural real strength.

Q. 71. If man is to grow up healthy and strong, how must he be educated.

A. He ought to receive a liberal, judicious, and prudent, education in his infancy, as well as in his youth.

Q. 72. Is this of so much importance?

A. Yes; for upon that depends his health, strength, and the happiness of his succeeding days.

Q. 73.

Q. 73. What is understood by a judicious education?

A. That man be educated agreeably with the nature of his soul and body.

Q. 74. What is, therefore, necessary to be known that we may give a judicious education to children?

A. The nature of man and of his existence?

Q. 75. What changes does man undergo during the first nine or twelve years of his existence?

A. His body grows and acquires shape; his soul learns the use of the body; his senses, with regard to conception and perception, increase; and he is joyful and happy in company with those of his own age.

Q. 76. What does nature particularly attempt to effect during infancy?

A. The formation of the body.

Q. 77. Is the energy of the soul, and the accomplishment of man, promoted by the perfection of the body?

A. Yes; the more perfect the body is the more perfect is the soul, and the more man is capable of promoting his own happiness, and that of his fellow-creatures.

Q. 78. Can the mind know the nature and structure of the body without instruction and labour?

A. No; the mind must for many years, during the whole period of infancy, study to acquire a thorough knowledge of the use of the body, composed of so many parts.

OBSERVATION.

All voluntary actions of the body are caused by about 440 muscles, which the mind puts in motion by means of a still greater number of nerves; the mind, therefore, during infancy, when we are full of life and vigour, and that the body is alert, must endeavour to learn the use of these 440 muscles, so as judiciously to call forth, as occasion may require, the various motions and energies of the body.

Q. 79. Are those motions or actions of any use to the body?

A. Yes;

A. Yes; its perfection is thereby promoted, and the whole body filled with life and vigour.

Q. 80. Of what use are those sensations and ideas to the child which its soul conceives through the senses?

A. They are the foundation of its understanding; for the more the mind has seen, heard, and felt, and the more distinct its sensations are, the more sensible will man become.

Q. 81. What particular purpose is answered by children living together?

A. They learn to know, to understand, and to love each other, and so lay a foundation for unanimity, mutual fondness, and the happiness of their lives.

Q. 82. But if children live in society merry and happy together, can that have any influence upon them when they arrive at a state of maturity?

A. Yes; it contributes very much to make man spend his life, according to his destination, in virtue and happiness.

Q. 83. By what means are those wise designs of Nature promoted?

A. By activity, and gentle, though constant exercise both of the mind and body of children.

Q. 84. Is such exercise compatible with the nature of children?

A. Yes; children are full of vigour and activity, sense and feeling; they are joyful and merry, and desire to associate with other children.

OBSERVATION.

From the twelfth to the eighteenth year the supple body should be invigorated by exercise and plays; the intuitive mind, by instruction and reflection, may lay up a store of knowledge, and man, whose infancy was passed in joy and happiness, learn to become virtuous in his youth; and he will become so if he has experienced the vicissitudes of fortune, her smiles and frowns, and shared his joys with others; if he firmly believes that

that all the defcendants of Adam have an equal right to enjoy pleafures, and are equally obnoxious to pain; and that an all-wife good God created every thing good, and mankind, with a view of making them happy.

Q. 85. What ought we further particularly to obferve with refpect to children?

A. That children be fuffered to exercife their bodies and minds in company with each other in the open air.

OBSERVATION.

Parents ought not only to be prefent at the exercifes and amufements of their children, and guard them from all dangers and injuries, but they ought alfo to encourage them, and lead them to all that is good and becoming, by their own virtuous example.

Q. 86. Ought female children to receive the fame education as boys in their infancy.

A. Yes; that they may at a future period enjoy the bleffings of perfect health as well as men.

OBSERVATION.

The moft pernicious confequences to the rifing generation flow from feparating female children, at the earlieft period of their exiftence, from male children; from dreffing them in a different manner, preventing them from taking the fame kind of exercife, and compelling them to lead a more fedentary life.

Q. 87. What are the confequences of preventing children from taking the neceffary exercifes before the ninth year?

A. Their growth is impeded, and they remain weak and fickly for life.

Q. 88. What effect will it have upon children if they are kept to too hard work before the twelfth year?

A. They will very foon grow ftiff, and old before their time.

VI. *Of*

VI. *Of Clothes fit to be worn by Children from the beginning of the Third to the End of the Seventh or Eighth Year; or till, in each of the two Jaws, the four weak Milk Teeth in Front are changed for four strong lasting Teeth.*

Q. 89. By what means does man preserve, particularly in his infancy, the genial warmth of his body?
A. By good wholesome food and bodily exercise.

Q. 90. Is it necessary to keep children warm, and protect them against the inclemency of the weather, by many garments?
A. No.

Q. 91. Why so?
A. That the body may grow healthy and strong, and be less liable to disease.

Q. 92. How ought the heads of children to be kept?
A. Clean and cool.

Q. 93. Is it good to cover childrens' heads with caps and hats to keep them warm?
A. No; it is very bad; the hair is a sufficient protection against cold.

Q. 94. Are those artificial coverings dangerous and hurtful?
A. Yes; children are thereby rendered simple and stupid, breed vermin, become scurfy, full of humours, and troubled with aches in their heads, ears, and teeth.

Q. 95. What kind of caps are, therefore, the most dangerous?
A. The woollen, cotton, and fur caps.

Q. 96. How, then, ought the heads of children to be kept?
A. Boys, as well as girls, ought to remain uncovered, winter or summer, by day and by night.

OBSERVATION.

OBSERVATION.

Children with scurfy heads ought to keep their heads cool, clean, and uncovered; their hair cut, or repeatedly combed; which will be sufficient to cure the evil, for to cure it with salves is a very dangerous custom.

Q. 97. Can the sun or air be prejudicial to the skin?

A. No; if proper care be taken to keep the skin clean, they can do no harm.

Q. 98. But will not children be scorched by the sun if exposed to its heat without being covered?

A. No; those that are accustomed from their infancy to go uncovered will not be affected by the sun.

Q. 99. How is the hair to be kept?

A. It ought not to be combed backwards, or tied behind; but it ought to hang free round the head to protect it.

Q. 100. Ought the hair to be often combed?

A. Yes; it ought to be kept in order and combed repeatedly every day; which prevents vermin from settling in it, and induces cheerfulness and liveliness.

Q. 101. Is it right that the collars of shirts and neckcloths should press the neck and its veins?

A. No; the neck ought not to be squeezed; and, therefore, children ought to have their necks bare.

Q. 102. How ought childrens' garments to be arranged?

A. So as not to impede the free and easy motions of the body, or prevent the access of the fresh strengthening air to it; they, therefore, ought to be free, wide, and open.

Q. 103. What further is requisite for this dress?

A. It ought to be simple, clean, light, cool, cheap, and easy to put on or take off; it ought to be different in every respect from that of older or grown-up persons.

Q. 104. What other reason is there for making this distinction between the dress of children and grown-up persons?

A. To

A. To induce children to live with lefs reftraint and greater happinefs in the fociety of each other; to imprefs upon their minds an idea of their weak, helplefs condition, in order thereby to check the too early ebullitions of that pride which leads children to ape the cuftoms and actions of grown-up perfons; a practice unbecoming at their age, and dangerous, perhaps, to their health and morals.

Q. 105. How, and of what materials, ought childrens' garments to be made?

A. A child ought to wear a wide linen frock, white, with blue ftripes, having wide fhort fleeves, and a fhirt of the fame form.

OBSERVATION.

The fhape of the frock is reprefented in the frontifpiece to this book; it ought to be without pocket-holes, and not very long, having the fleeves of fufficient length to reach down to the elbows, and no farther. The collar of the fhirt to fall back over that of the frock,—the only garment that a child fhould wear over his fhirt, in order that it may move eafily and without reftraint; and that the frefh air, having free accefs to its body, may ftrengthen and invigorate it.

Q. 106. Ought children to wear this drefs in the winter time?

A. Yes; with the addition of a woollen frock, to be worn between the fhirt and the linen frock.

Q. 107. How are the ftockings of children to be made?

A. They muft be fhort, and not tied; it would, therefore, be advifeable to let them only wear focks, to cover the feet in the fhoes.

OBSERVATION.

Stockings that cover the knees may produce fwellings in them; they ought, therefore, not to cover the knees, nor be worn with garters.

Q. 108.

[27]

Q. 108. Will not children find themselves too cold if their ankles are left bare?

A. No; cold, if they are accustomed to it, will not affect their ankles more than their arms. It will strengthen their limbs. In short they will be kept sufficiently warm by the shirt and frock.

OBSERVATION.

In England children wear no stockings at all, or only socks.

Q. 109. What is the form of the human foot?
A. At the toes it is broad, the heel small, and the inside of the foot is longer than the outside. See Fig. I.

Q. 110. Why has it this form?
A. That man may walk and stand with ease and firmness, and move his body freely.

Q. 111. How ought shoes, particularly those of children, to be formed?
A. They ought to have the same form as the feet; they, therefore, ought not to be made by one, but two lasts, as the shape of the feet may indicate.

OBSERVATION.

Each foot may be laid upon a sheet of paper, and its true shape drawn with a pencil, after which model two separate lasts may be made.

From the following figures it appears clearly how shoes ought to be shaped. The middle Fig. I. is the original shape of the sole of the left foot; the first, Fig. III shows how the sole of the left shoe ought to be formed; and the last Fig. II. shows clearly, that the shoes we usually wear, made on one last, do not at all fit.

Fig. III.

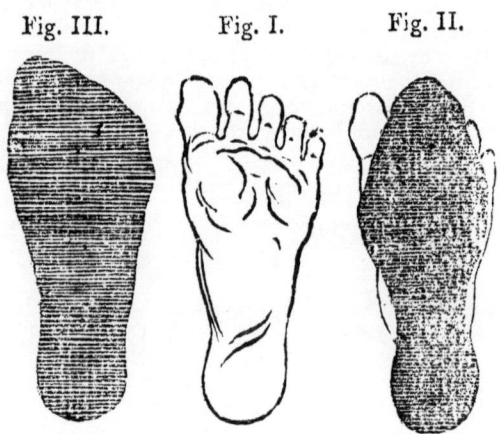

Fig. III. Fig. I. Fig. II.

Q. 112. Ought the shoes of children to have heels?

A. No; heels cause the back-bone to bend, and impede the free and easy motions of the body in walking and running.

OBSERVATION.

In order to obtain or preserve an upright posture or carriage of the body, and to run and jump easily and conveniently, shoes without heels must be worn.

When children are suffered to walk much, and are barefooted, they acquire an easy and steady pace. Little children ought not to wear shoes before the eighteenth month; if they do the soles must be thin and soft, that they may learn to walk easily and well. Boots ought not to be worn by children.

Q. 113. How ought, therefore, children, male as well as female, to be dressed from the beginning of the third to the end of the seventh or eighth year?

A. Their

A. Their heads and necks muſt be free and bare, the body clothed with a wide ſhirt and frock, with ſhort ſleeves; the feet covered only with a pair of ſocks to be worn in the ſhoes; the ſhoes ought to be made without heels, and to fit well.

Q. 114. What benefit will be derived from this kind of dreſs?

A. The body will become healthier, ſtronger, taller, and more beautiful; children will learn the beſt and moſt graceful attitudes; and will feel themſelves very well and happy in this ſimple and free garment.

OBSERVATION.

That by the general introduction of this ſimple and eaſy dreſs, the human race would be benefited and rendered every way more accompliſhed, it cannot be doubted. It is, therefore, to be hoped that it will be generally adopted.

Q. 115. How muſt the whole dreſs be kept?

A. Orderly and clean. The ſhirt ought always to be clean, and the frock decent, not worn out, or torn to pieces, or unclean.

Q. 116. When children appear always combed and waſhed, and in a clean ſhirt, and dreſſed from top to toe with decency and cleanlineſs, what is commonly concluded from it?

A. That their parents are ſenſible, kind, and loving.

Q. 117. And with reſpect to the children themſelves?

A. They are beloved: the boy will become a worthy man, the girl an excellent wife; and both imitate the example of their parents.

Q. 118. Is it proper that grown-up perſons, but, eſpecially, is it proper that children, ſhould be dreſſed in an oſtentatious manner, or ſhew any pride in their attire?

A. No; ſimple, decent, clean, eaſy dreſs is the beſt.

Eccleſiaſticus

Ecclesiasticus x. 7. Pride is hateful before God and man; and by both doth one commit iniquity.

OBSERVATION.

> Stays and stiff jackets are inventions of the most pernicious nature; they disfigure the beautiful and upright shape of a woman, and, instead of rendering her straight, as was formerly supposed, they make her crooked-backed; they injure the breasts and bowels; obstruct the breathing and digestion; hurt the breasts and nipples so much, that many mothers are prevented by their use from suckling their children; many hence get cancers, and at last lose both health and life; they in general destroy health, and render the delivery of women very difficult and dangerous both to mother and child.
> It is, therefore, the duty of parents, and especially of mothers, to banish from their houses and families both stays and jackets. Those girdles or sashes which press or constrain the belly are equally injurious; and, in general, it would be a desirable thing, if the female dress were made to consist of a long, easy, and beautiful robe, and not of two parts, joining or meeting at the hips.

Q. 119. Is it adviseable to wear clothes that have been worn by people who were infected by epidemic disorders, or who died thereof; or to make dresses of them for children?

A. No; it might cause an entire loss of health, and, perhaps, life.

OBSERVATION.

> Old clothes, particularly old woollen clothes, infected by unwholesome perspiration, are very injurious to health, and epidemic fevers are hence easily and frequently propagated.

THE following Chapters regard grown-up persons as much as children; those parts alluding to the latter only, will be pointed out in particular queries and answers.

VII. Of Air.

Q. 120. WHAT ought to be the state of the air in which man liveth, and every moment breathes?

A. The air in which man liveth, and which he breathes, ought to be fresh, clear, and dry.

Q. 121. Why ought it to be fresh, clear, and dry?

A. Because it tends to refresh us, and makes us healthy, composed, and serene; it encourages man to work cheerfully, excites appetite, improves health, and induces balmy sleep; in short, man finds himself exceedingly happy while he breathes fresh air.

Q. 122. Does he feel equally as comfortable when he breathes bad, foul, and damp air?

A. No: in bad corrupted air man becomes weak, unhealthy, and irritable; loathsome and stupid; it often causes fevers and many dangerous maladies very difficult to cure.

Q. 123. Is it very necessary that man should live in fresh air, in order to enjoy a perfect state of health?

A. As unavoidably necessary as eating and drinking: as clean water is to fishes.

Q. 124. Why is it so?

A. Because the ambient air contains, as well as our food, vital principles, very peculiar ones, which cannot be dispensed with, or supplied by any thing except the air we breathe.

OBSERVATION.

Even plants in the best soil, and beasts receiving the most wholesome food, will decay without good pure air. Man, therefore, in particular, requires

requires fresh air, that he may live and thrive, be healthy, sensible, serene, and happy.

Q. 125. By what means is air corrupted?

A. The air is corrupted in houses and rooms that are not sufficiently ventilated: beside, if in the vicinity of the habitations of man there be morasses, or stagnant waters, they are sufficient to corrupt the circumambient air.

Q. 126. By what other means is air rendered obnoxious?

A. Vapours arising from damp, foul things; the breath and perspiration of many persons; the smoke from lamps, tallow-candles, and snuffs; the steam from ironing linen; the exhalations that arise from combing wool, and from burning charcoal; all tend, in a greater or lesser degree, to corrupt or deprave the atmosphere, and render it capable of impeding the action of the lungs, or inducing suffocation.

Q. 127. What ought people to do that are much confined to rooms or chambers?

A. They ought frequently to open their doors and windows, in order to dissipate corrupted air, and admit the cooling, healthful zephyrs.

Q. 128. What other method can be devised to prevent the depravation of air in a room.

A. By making two holes, one through the outer wall of the house, that will open into the room near the floor of it; the other near the cieling, through the opposite inner wall or partition; the external atmosphere will enter at the hole near the floor, and dissipate the foul air through the aperture above.

Q. 129. What else ought people to do, to obtain so desirable an end?

A. They ought to keep their rooms or apartments clean, and in proper order; nothing superfluous, or that can possibly corrupt the air, ought to be suffered in them.

OBSERVATION.

Perfumes, and flowers emitting a strong smell, are very dangerous in rooms, particularly in bed-chambers;

chambers; they corrupt the air, and cause headach, giddiness, and sometimes apoplexy.

Q. 130. What are the signs by which you may know whether rooms be clean, and contain wholesome air?

A. When there are no cob-webs in the corners, or on the cieling, of the room, nor dust, nor straw, nor filth of any kind; when the windows are clean and clear, and that no offensive smell, or unpleasant sensation, is experienced by a person who enters it that has been just breathing the open air, we conclude that it is as it ought to be.

Q. 131. Is it necessary for man to breathe fresh air when asleep?

A. Yes: It is necessary that he breathe good wholesome air, whether awake or asleep: curtains encompassing a bed, and narrow bed-steads, are therefore very unwholesome.

OBSERVATION.

To cover childrens' faces when they are asleep is a bad custom, for they are thereby deprived of fresh air.

Q. 132. If people that are much confined to their rooms were careful to live always in fresh air, what would be the natural consequence?

A. Instead of being unhealthy, weak, and squalid, and labouring under catarrh, cold, and hoarseness, they would be much more healthy, content, and happy, and live longer.

OBSERVATION.

To bury the dead in or near towns and villages is very injurious and dangerous to the living.

VIII. *Of Cleanliness:—Washing and Bathing.*

Q. 133. OF what use is cleanliness to man?

A. It preserves his health and virtue; it clears his understanding,

understanding, and encourages him to activity; it procures him the esteem of others; and none but clean people can be really cheerful and happy.

Q. 134. How far is uncleanliness injurious to man?

A. It corrupts his health and virtue; it stupifies his mind, and sinks it into a lethargic state; it deprives him of the esteem and love of others; beside, unclean people can never be really merry and happy.

Q. 135. Does uncleanliness cause any maladies?

A. Yes. Uncleanliness and bad air, which are commonly inseparable, produce fevers, which are not only very malignant and mortal, but contagious also.

OBSERVATION.

Doctor Ferriar of Manchester, so renowned for his humanity, proves from the epidemical poison which commonly originates in the huts of misery, that not only virtue and charity, but also self-preservation, point out to the rich that it is their duty to relieve the poor.

Q. 136. What impels man most to keep himself clean?

A. The being accustomed from his infancy to cleanliness in his person, his dress, and habitation.

Q. 137. What must be done to keep the body clean?

A. It is not sufficient to wash the face, hands, and feet; it is also necessary, more than once, and at short intervals, to wash the skin all over the body, and to bathe frequently.

Q. 138. Is washing and bathing the whole body wholesome?

A. Yes, it is very good; for it begets cleanliness, health, strength, and ease; and prevents catarrhs, cramps, rheumatism, palsy, the itch, and many other maladies.

OBSERVATION.

In Russia almost every house has its bath; and it were to be wished that each village or town in every

every country contained one or more houses, where people might be accommodated with cold and warm baths.

Q. 139. Why is the keeping the body so clean of so great importance?

A. Because the half of whatever man eats or drinks is evacuated by perspiration; and if the skin is not kept clean, the pores are stopped and perspiration consequently prevented, to the great injury of health.

Q. 140. What rules are to be observed with respect to bathing?

A. 1. That you be careful to bathe in places where you are not exposed to danger.

2. That you feel yourself thoroughly well and in good health, and that you be not over-heated at the time of going into the bath, which should not be immediately after a repast.

3. That you go not into the bath slowly, and by degrees, but plunge in all at once.

4. That after bathing you repose not, but walk about leisurely.

OBSERVATION.

It would be very adviseable to impel scholars to bathe, under the inspection of their masters, a certain number of times each week, from the beginning of May, till the end of September.

Q. 141. How often is it necessary to wash hands and face?

A. In the morning, and going to rest; before and after dinner and supper, and as often as they are by any means soiled.

OBSERVATION.

In each regular house there ought to be constantly ready a wash-hand bason, and clear cold water, for that purpose.

Q. 142. Is it not necessary after meals to clean or wash the mouth?

A. Yes.

A. Yes. Immediately after each repaſt the mouth ought to be cleanſed with cold water; the gums and teeth are thus preſerved ſound and good, and the tooth-ach prevented.

Q. 143. Ought not children to be waſhed and combed before they go to ſchool?

A. Yes. Children ought, morning and evening, before they go to ſchool, to be combed and waſhed; that, being thus rendered comfortable and cheerful, they may with greater eaſe and pleaſure advance in the paths of ſcience and virtue.

Q. 144. What ought you particularly to do when you waſh yourſelf?

A. We ought always to immerſe our faces in the water, and keep them ſo for a little time.

OBSERVATION.

Thus we accuſtom ourſelves to reſtrain our breath, which in caſe of danger in the water will be found of great uſe. And if we open our eyes in the water, and clean the mouth, it will prove beneficial to both, and prevent tooth-ach.

Q. 145. As it is neceſſary that the body ſhould be kept clean from the earlieſt infancy, and as little children are not capable of waſhing and attending themſelves, what duty is therefore impoſed upon parents?

A. It is as much their duty to waſh their children as it is to feed and cloath them; for children that are often waſhed improve in health; their clothes are always clean; cleanlineſs becomes familiar to them; and they grow up virtuous, polite, and happy.

Q. 146. Do little children like to be bathed and waſhed?

A. In the beginning they are frightened, and cry; but if they be regularly and frequently bathed, and often waſhed every day, they at laſt take delight in it.

Q. 147. Is it ſufficient that man keep his body clean?

A. No. He muſt alſo keep his clothes clean, and all that is about him; his apartments, beds, and furniture: and they ought alſo to be kept in order.

Q. 148

Q. 148. What benefit doth the whole household derive from such order and cleanliness?

A. It tends to preserve their health; makes all work easy, and renders life joyous and happy.

IX. *Of Food.*

Q. 149. WHY doth man eat?
A. To satisfy the cravings of hunger, to preserve life, and to nourish the body.

Q. 150. What kind of food doth man generally partake of?
A. Bread, vegetables, fruit, milk, fish, and meat.

Q. 151. Which of these yields the greatest nourishment?
A. Meat, or animal food, which is more nourishing than vegetables.

Q. 152. Of what ought our meals to consist?
A. Chiefly of vegetables.

OBSERVATION.

That man was not designed to live on meat, or on vegetables, only, is evident from the construction of his teeth, his stomach, and bowels. Living upon animal food only causes putrefaction of the blood; and vegetables by themselves do not sufficiently nourish or strengthen the body.

Q. 153. What gives the most delicious relish to food?
A. Hunger, and the thorough mastication of the food.

Q. 154. What tends most to promote hunger and digestion.
A. Bodily exercise, especially in the open air.

Q. 155. Is it best to eat simple food?
A. Yes. It is destructive of health to partake of many different dishes, or of such as are prepared with
much

much art; for they are very difficult of digeftion, and afford bad and unwholefome nourifhment.

Q. 156. What is particularly to be obferved at meals?

A. Order and moderation; and that the food be well mafticated, in order that it may the more readily be converted into chyle.

OBSERVATION.

By maftication the teeth are kept found and faft. It is therefore neceffary to make children chew on both fides of the mouth.

Q. 157. What does Sirach fay of frugality?

A. Ecclefiafticus xxxi. 20. he fays, " Sound fleep " cometh of moderate eating: he rifeth early, and " his wits are with him: but the pains of watching, " and choler, and pangs of the belly, are with an " unfatiable man."

Q. 158. If our food be not fufficiently mafticated and converted into a pap-like fubftance, what is the confequence?

A. It cannot be digefted fufficiently; and undigefted food yields bad nourifhment to the body—overloads the ftomach, and induces a weak, morbid ftate of the fyftem.

Q. 159. Is it good to drink much at meals?

A. No. Too much drink renders our food too fluid.

Q. 160. Does fluid aliment afford wholefome and ftrong nourifhment?

A. No. Food of whatever kind, in order that it may afford proper nourifhment, ought to be fubftantial: it is therefore neceffary to eat bread with fluid aliment.

OBSERVATION.

Even the milk which the child fucks muft firft curdle in the ftomach before it can give any nourifhment to the body.

Q. 161. As bread is our principal food, what ought to be its appropriate qualities?

A. It

A. It ought to be made from good corn, and well baked.

OBSERVATION.

Westphalian pumpernickel, or black bread, is, for healthy, strong, hard labouring people, a good wholesome kind of food; but it is too heavy for children, aged persons, or such as lead a sedentary life, and yields them but little nourishment.

Q. 162. What must we have to be able to bake good bread?

A. 1. Clean and dry corn, that is not damp, musty, or in a state of vegetation.

2. Flour that has not fermented in the sacks or boxes.

3. Too much, or too hard water, is not to be used; but soft water may be employed for making the dough, which requires to be well kneaded.

4. Fresh good yeast is required.

5. The leavened dough ought to swell considerably in a temperate heat, and

6. The oven ought not to be too cold, nor too hot.

Q. 163. If rye be mixed with much cockle-seed, mother-wort, or other tare-seed, will make it wholesome bread?

A. No. It makes bad and unwholesome bread.

Q. 164. If rye be damp, musty, or in a state of vegetation; or if it has grown in a wet season, ought bread to be made of it?

A. No. It is very dangerous to eat such bread; for it induces sickness and anxiety; and frequently begets contagious and putrid fevers, which lay waste whole provinces.

Q. 165. How can such damp, bad rye or corn be improved so far as that wholesome bread may be made of it?

A. The corn ought to be dried before it is ground, and the bad flour mixed with some good orris, rye, or barley flour: a little water, in which a certain quantity of pot-ash has been dissolved, may be made use of to moisten it; the bread must be baked slowly and well,

well, and muſt not be eaten when warm or new, nor in too a great a quantity.

OBSERVATION.

Children ought to be carefully inſtructed how to make good wholeſome bread, how to preſerve good corn, and to correct that which has been ſpoiled. There is a compendious little book on this ſubject; it is generally read in Germany. As it contains many uſeful and intereſting inſtructions reſpecting perſons who have been drowned or poiſoned, or who have met with other accidents, it will ſoon be tranſlated and offered to the public.

Q. 166. Is hot bread or cakes wholeſome?
A. No. They are very unwholeſome: they may cauſe ſickneſs and death.

Q. 167. Potatoes, when eaten in moderation, are good and wholeſome; but, do they prove ſalutary when eaten in too great quantity, and every day?
A. No. Potatoes eaten every day and in great quantity, are not very wholeſome; they afford ſcanty nouriſhment.

OBSERVATION.

Potatoes, when eaten too often, or immoderately, prove hurtful to health, and to the mental faculties.

Q. 168. What is further to be obſerved with reſpect to potatoes?
A. Potatoes ought not to be eaten before they are quite ripe; and care ſhould be taken that they do not grow muſty, or ſhoot out in damp cellars—ſuch potatoes are bad.

OBSERVATION.

As potatoes degenerate that are year after year dug from the old roots, and loſe their ʼpriſtine virtues, it would be beſt that part of the potatoes be be eaten this year, and part be kept for feed for the next, and so on; which will produce much finer and more wholesome potatoes than the others.

Q. 169. Are ripe fruits and acid substances wholesome?

A. Yes: they cleanse and refresh the body.

OBSERVATION.

With respect to the kernels of fruits, children ought to be cautioned not to swallow them, as they may cause an obstruction in the bowels and consequent death.

Q. 170. Are fat meats wholesome? and is it good to give much bread and butter to children?

A. No; it is not good. Bread and butter, like all fat aliments, are difficult of digestion; they are prejudicial to health, generate a great deal of bile, and produce worms.

OBSERVATION.

All children, without exception, have naturally worms in their bowels; but those worms are only hurtful and dangerous, when, from bad, indigestible food, and want of exercise, the bowels are over-loaded with slime, which disposes to the generation of worms.

Q. 171. Are astringent, salted, or high-seasoned viands wholesome?

A. No; they are unwholesome; and children ought not to eat astringent, pickled, or high-seasoned meats.

Q. 172. What is in general to be observed with respect to the feeding of children?

A. They ought to be fed regularly every day at stated times, and often; their food ought to be mild and nourishing, that they may grow and thrive well.

Q. 173. Is it good to give children dainties, cakes, or sweetmeats?

A. No. Children are thereby rendered too fond of their bellies, become gluttons, and degenerate from the dignity of their nature.

OBSERVATION.

> Sweetmeats, and all the toys of children, are commonly covered with poisonous paint: they therefore ought to be prohibited.

Q. 174. What is the state of the kitchen of a good orderly wife or house-keeper?

A. The kitchen furniture is always kept clean by scouring and washing; after any part of it has been used, it is immediately washed, and dried with a clean cloth, and put up in its proper place; and when it is wanted again, it is first of all dusted and rubbed well.

Q. 175. What is especially to be observed with respect to the preparing and keeping of victuals?

A. The greatest cleanliness; and the eatables ought neither to be prepared nor kept in improper vessels, or such as can communicate to them any poisonous quality.

Q. 176. Ought every thing first to be washed before it is boiled or roasted?

A. Yes. Every kind of food, whether animal or vegetable, ought to well washed before it is boiled or roasted; and vegetables especially require washing to remove mildew or insects.

Q. 177. What sort of kitchen utensils may become noxious?

A. Those of copper, which are not perfectly well tinned, and earthen vessels which are glazed with too much lead.

OBSERVATION.

> Earthen vessels receive a varnish of sand and prepared lead; if too much of the latter be used, or if the varnish be not well burnt, acids will dissolve

dissolve the lead, and render it capable of communicating a deleterious impregnation to food.

Q. 178. If acescent food, especially, be prepared and kept, or suffered to cool, in such vessels, what are the consequences?

A. It dissolves and mixes with part of the lead or copper, and so becomes capable, if eaten, of producing gradual loss of health: sudden death may be the unavoidable consequence.

Q. 179. What is therefore to be observed with respect to those vessels?

A. Those of copper ought to be well tinned; the earthen ones must have a very hard and durable varnish, consisting of but little lead, and ought to be well seasoned by keeping them a proper time immersed in boiling water, in which pot-ashes have been dissolved; and neither the copper nor the earthen vessels ought to be used for cooling or keeping victuals.

Q. 180. Are pewter vessels also dangerous in this respect?

A. They are. Pewter is often mixed with a great deal of lead; and therefore victuals ought not to be kept in vessels of this kind.

Q. 181. What kind of water ought to be used for the boiling of victuals?

A. Not only for boiling victuals, but for baking and brewing, clean soft water is required, in which dry peas can be boiled soft.

X. *On Drink.*

Q. 182. FOR what purpose is it necessary that man should drink?

A. To quench his thirst; but not to gratify his palate, or to strengthen his stomach, or with a view hence to derive nourishment; for all such notions are wrong, and against nature.

Q. 183.

Q. 183. What kind of beverage therefore is the moſt proper?

A. Cold water.

Q. 184. What advantage do we derive from drinking cold water?

A. Cold water cools, thins, and clears the blood; it keeps the ſtomach, bowels, head, and nerves in order, and makes man tranquil, ſerene, and cheerful.

Q. 185. What is it that gives to cold water an agreeable taſte, and renders it nouriſhing?

A. Bodily exerciſe in the open air not only induces thirſt, and a deſire for water, but alſo renders it nouriſhing.

OBSERVATION.

By the movement of the body, water is cauſed to mix thoroughly with the blood, whoſe viſcid, ſharp, and acrid humours it expels from the body.

Q. 186. Do people commonly drink a ſufficient quantity of cold water?

A. No. Many, from not taking ſufficient exerciſe in the open air, and from drinking frequently large quantities of warm drink, loſe all real thirſt; and, from not drinking a ſufficient quantity of cold water, their blood remains viſcid, acrid, and impure.

OBSERVATION.

Females, in particular, that are much confined at home, drink a great deal of coffee and tea, but do not drink enough of cold water.

Q. 187. May we drink any water without diſtinction?

A. No. We ought not to drink ſtagnant, unclean, muddy, or putrefied water.

OBSERVATION.

If one be under the unavoidable neceſſity of drinking bad or foul water, a little vinegar may be mixed

mixed with it, which is the beft corrector of it.

Q. 188. What kind of water is beft for drinking?

A. Pure, clear water, without tafte, fmell, or colour;—water in which foap will readily diffolve, and peas readily foften, if boiled in it.

OBSERVATION.

The old Romans made aqueducts of fuch a length, that five, ten, or more hours, would be confumed in walking from one extremity to the other of fome of them; and they did fo in order to furnifh populous places with good wholefome water for drinking.

Q. 189. Is beer a wholefome beverage?

A. Light, well-brewed beer is not injurious to the health of grown-up perfons; though certainly good water is much better, and more wholefome.

OBSERVATION.

Children, by drinking beer, lofe the defire of drinking water, and fo fteal into the habit of drinking too much coffee, tea, wine, and brandy.

Q. 190. Are warm drinks, fuch as coffee, tea, &c. wholefome?

A. No. The only wholefome beverage is cold water; all warm drinks weaken the ftomach and body; they do not cleanfe the bowels, nor purify the blood, and are, therefore, unwholefome and hurtful to health.

Q. 191. Why are people, particularly females, fo fond of tea and coffee?

A. Becaufe, for want of exercife, they have no natural or real thirft; and becaufe they have been ufed to them from their infancy.

OBSERVATION.

If water were the only drink of man, both his health and fortune would be improved. If what is fpent on fluids that are hurtful to life were
appropriated

appropriated to the purchafe of nourifhing food, and other neceffaries of life, the lot of humankind would be meliorated, and we fhould live longer, and be healthier, ftronger, and happier.

Q. 192. What, then, ought to be the only beverage for children?

A. Pure, good cold water ought to be the only drink of children and young folks; who ought to be prohibited from drinking beer, coffee, tea, or other warm liquors.

Q. 193. What advantage do children and young perfons derive from drinking cold water only?

A. They grow, and are nourifhed, much better, and become healthier, ftronger, and happier.

XI. *Of Wine.*

Q. 194. Is wine wholefome, when drank often, or as a common beverage?

A. No; it is not. Wine is very hurtful to the health, the intellects, and the happinefs of man.

Q. 195. Wine, as a medical potion, comforts the fick, and ftrengthens the weak; but does it afford any real ftrength or nourifhment to the healthy?

A. No; it only over-heats, without procuring real ftrength; for it cannot be converted into good blood, flefh, or bone.

Q. 196. Does wine contribute to the digeftion of our meals?

A. No; it does not. Thofe that drink water eat with a better appetite, and digeft better, than thofe that drink wine.

Q. 197. What confequences enfue from drinking wine continually?

A. The tongue lofes its delicacy of tafte, and rejects water and mild fimple food; the ftomach grows cold and lofes its natural vigour, and man, under the falfe idea of giving warmth to his ftomach, gains by degrees

degrees a paffion for drinking, which leads him at laſt to habitual ebriety.

OBSERVATION.

Young and bad wines, full of impure, earthy parts, and volatile ſpirit, are much more hurtful than old wines of a good vintage. Wine adulterated with any preparation of lead, as ſugar of lead, white lead, &c. is poiſon.

Q. 198. May children drink wine, punch, or other ſpirituous intoxicating liquors?
A. No. Children and young perſons ought not to drink wine, or any other ſpirituous liquors; for they are hurtful to health, impede growth, obſcure reaſon, and lay a foundation for wretchedneſs hereafter.

Q. 199. Does wine expel worms?
A. No; it does not.

XII. *Of Brandy.*

OBSERVATION.

VEGETATION has united and incorporated in the corn, by means of air and water, ſpirituous and earthy elements, which combined form a ſweet and nouriſhing ſubſtance; if this intimate junction is deſtroyed or reſolved by fermentation, the ſpirituous part is ſeparated from the earthy, which is then deprived of its body, and is no longer a ſweet nouriſhing ſubſtance, it is fiery, and deſtroys like fire.

Q. 200. Is brandy a good liquor?
A. No.

ADDRESS TO CHILDREN.

Children, brandy is a bad liquor. A few hundred years ago brandy was not known among us. About 1000 years ago, the deſtructive art of diſtilling
ſpirits

spirits of wine from wine was found out; and 300 years ago, brandy was firſt diſtilled from corn. In the beginning it was conſidered as phyſic. It did not, however, gain any degree of general requeſt till the cloſe of the laſt century, or rather till within the laſt thirty years, that it has become an univerſal beverage, to the great detriment of mankind.

Our forefathers in former times, who had no idea of brandy, were quite different people from what we are; they were much more healthy and ſtrong. Brandy, whether drank by itſelf or at meals, cannot be converted into blood, fleſh, or bone; conſequently, it cannot give health or ſtrength, nor does it promote digeſtion: it only makes one unhealthy, ſtupid, lazy, and weak. It is, therefore, a downright falſehood, that brandy, as a common beverage, is uſeful, good, and neceſſary. Our forefathers lived without it. And as experience teaches us, that even the moſt moderate and moſt reaſonable give way to the baneful cuſtom of drinking every day more and more brandy, it is much better, in order to avoid temptation, to drink none at all; for, believe me, children, brandy deprives every body who addicts himſelf to the immoderate and daily uſe of it—of health, reaſon, and virtue. It impels us to quit our houſe and home, and to abandon our wives and children, and entails on its wretched votaries miſery and diſeaſe, which may deſcend to the third and fourth generation.

It has been obſerved in all countries, in England, Scotland, Sweden, North America, and Germany, that in proportion to the quantity of brandy conſumed, were the evils which health, ſtrength, reaſon, virtue, induſtry, proſperity, domeſtic and matrimonial felicity, the education of children, humanity, and the life of man had to encounter.

It was this that induced an Indian in North America, of the name of Lackawanna, to ſay, that
the

the brandy which had been introduced amongſt the Indians by the Engliſh, tended to corrupt mankind and deſtroy humanity. " They have " given us (ſaid he) brandy ! and who has given " it to them (Europeans), who elſe but an evil " ſpirit !"

Q. 201. Tell me, therefore, dear children, may children drink brandy?

A. No, by no means; children muſt not only abſtain from brandy, but alſo from rum, gin, and all other ſpirituous liquors.

ADMONITION.

It is true that children muſt not drink brandy, not even a ſingle drop, for brandy deprives children of their health and reaſon, of their virtue and happineſs. When, therefore, dear children, your parents, who, perhaps, do not know that brandy corrupts both body and ſoul, ſhall offer you any ſpirituous liquor, do not accept it, do not drink it.

Q. 202. Tell me now, what becomes of children that drink ſpirituous liquors?

A. Children and young perſons who drink brandy, or other ſpirituous liquors, become unhealthy, crippled, ſtupid, rude, lazy, vicious, and depraved, both as to mind and body.

Q. 203. Doth brandy, or any other ſpirituous liquor, deſtroy, or prevent, the generation of worms in the bowels?

A. No.

EXHORTATION.

Fathers and mothers, if you wiſh to obtain the bleſſing of the Almighty in an eſpecial manner—if you aſpire after celeſtial rewards, take care not to ſuffer your children to drink of ſpirituous liquors a ſingle drop.

E   XIII. *Of*

XIII. *Of Tobacco.*

Q. 204. IS the smoking of tobacco good?
A. No; it is not good, for much of the saliva so necessary for digestion is thereby lost, and it is hurtful to health, to the teeth, and to the organs of taste.

OBSERVATION.

The chewing of tobacco is equally pernicious.

Q. 205. May children and young people smoke tobacco?
A. No; children and youth must not smoke at all.

Q. 206. Is the taking of snuff proper?
A. No; it is a very bad custom, as the nose through which man breathes is stuffed up by it, the important sense of smell destroyed, and uncleanliness and want of health induced by its use.

XIV. *Of Exercise and Rest.*

Q. 207. WHAT advantage doth man derive from bodily exercise, activity, and labour?
A. Bodily exercise particularly in the open air, creates hunger and thirst, helps the digestion of our food, and makes it nourishing; it purifies the blood, keeps the bowels healthy, and causes rest and sound sleep.

Ecclesiasticus xxx. 18. " To labour and to be con-
" tent with that a man hath is a sweet life, but he
" that findeth a treasure is above them both."

Q. 208. Can any body remain in a good state of health, without much bodily exercise?
A. No; God has given to man, not without a wise design, a body, hands, and feet: he is to make use of them and labour, and through labour to preserve
life

life and health, to promote his own happiness, and that of his fellow-creatures.

Q. 209. But cannot exercise and labour hurt a man?

A. By all means: If man exceeds the bounds of reason, and of his natural powers, he may hurt himself.

OBSERVATION.

It is computed that, in Germany, 300,000 persons of the male sex are afflicted with ruptures.— What is the reason that people are so liable to ruptures? I believe I have proved satisfactorily, that ruptures will be far less frequent, will scarcely be met with, when the custom of dressing male children in frocks, such as I have described, is introduced, and that the muscles and nerves of the abdomen are strengthened by unrestrained exercise and fresh air. If he works continually and too hard, his body will be debilitated and worn out, or a rupture may be the fatal consequence.

Q. 210. Is it good to take much exercise, or work hard immediately before or after dinner?

A. No; a little rest before and after dinner is necessary, and promotes appetite and digestion, recruits the powers of the body, and fits it for future work.

Q. 211. What kind of exercise is proper for children?

A. Gentle and continued exercise in the open air, during the greater part of the day.

OBSERVATION.

The pulsations in a child are ninety in a minute; those in a man seventy. A child ought, therefore, to take a great deal of exercise of the gentlest kind. It is therefore not good to oblige children to lead a sedentary life, or to do too much or too heavy work, or study hard; after the shedding of the teeth the twelfth year, when they have twenty-four strong teeth, when soul and body have acquired their perfect strength and vigour, the time of instruction and work should begin, but not before, lest mind and body be injured.

Q. 212. How doth man become very active and industrious?

A. By being left during his childhood to exercise, unrestrained, with other children, and by being carefully encouraged to activity, assiduity, industry, and thinking; by being taught to do such work as is proportioned to the strength of his body, and accustomed to do every thing with due consideration and in time, and not to postpone till to-morrow, what should be done to-day.

Ecclesiasticus ix. 10. "Whatsoever thy hand "findeth to do, do it with thy might; for there is no "work, nor device, nor knowledge, nor wisdom, in "the grave, whither thou goest."

Q. 213. What advantages arise from accustoming children to moderate or easy work?

A. It renders them, when grown up, useful to themselves and their fellow-creatures; it will prevent them from mixing in bad company, and will banish want and misery from their doors.

Prov. x. 4. "He becometh poor that dealeth with "a slack hand, but the hand of the diligent maketh "rich."

Q. 214. After man has laboured, and finished his work, what then doth he do?

A. He rests himself, and looks with pleasure upon the fruits of his industry.

Q. 215. But would he rest as well if he had not laboured, or had not been industrious?

A. No. Peace, rest, and joy, are the exclusive enjoyments of him who has done his duty, who has worked and promoted his own, and the happiness of his fellow-creatures.

ADMONITION, OR ADDRESS TO CHILDREN.

Dear children! he who owes his birth and education to healthy, strong, sensible, virtuous, and industrious

industrious parents, who, from his infancy, has constantly inspired fresh, pure, and dry air; whose skin and apparel are always kept clean; who, with regard to his meals, observes moderation and order, and drinks no brandy or other spirituous liquors; whose habitation is orderly, clean, dry, and lightsome; who has been accustomed from his infancy to order and cleanliness, to assiduity and industry, and whose reason and virtue have been fortified and improved in his youth by instruction and example; who fears God, loves mankind, and does justice; who works six days out of seven for the maintenance of his wife and children:—he only enjoys terrestrial bliss; he is truly happy, and may, anticipating the joys of eternal felicity, brave all the horrors of death.

XV. *Of Sleep.*

Q. 216. FOR what purpose doth man go to sleep?
A. To rest himself after exercise and labour, and regain the strength of his body, and the faculties of his mind.

Q. 217. How do the healthy rest?
A. Their rest is quiet, refreshing, and without dreams.

Q. 218. When especially do the healthy enjoy a quiet and refreshing sleep?
A. When their bodies are wearied by much exercise in the open air; when they have satisfied hunger, and that their minds enjoy contentment and peace.

Q. 219 Doth much depend upon a sound sleep?
A. Yes; man after a night's balmy sleep awakes with delight and cheerfulness, finds himself quite happy, and full of vigour and desire for labour.

Q. 220. What time is particularly appropriated or sleep?

A. The

A. The night; for in the day-time we do not sleep so well.

OBSERVATION.

Little children, and people who are either sick or enfeebled, or very much tired, and the old and infirm, are to be excepted, as they very often sleep in the day-time.

Q. 221. Ought children to sleep much?

A. Yes; children and young people that are constantly in motion, ought to sleep more than adults.

Q. 222. Cannot we sleep too much, and so injure our health?

A. Yes: when we have not had much exercise in the open air, and consequently are not tired, and when we, during our sleep, breathe corrupted air, or lie in warm feather-beds, we find ourselves after some time lazy, stupid, and unhealthy.

Q. 223. Ought we to sleep in cool, fresh, and clear air?

A. Yes. And it therefore behoves us not to sleep in warm sitting rooms, but in cold, lofty, roomy chambers, that have fresh air; whose windows are kept open in the day-time, and contain beds without curtains, or curtains not to be drawn.

Q. 224. Is it wholesome to lay on, or under feather-beds?

A. No. It is very unwholesome. Feather-beds by their warmth, by the noxious, impure, putrid exhalations which they attract, render the body weak and unhealthy; and besides, are the cause of catarrhs, head, tooth, and ear, aches—of rheumatism, and of many other maladies.

Q. 225. What kind of bed is fittest for grown-up persons?

A. Mattresses stuffed with horse-hair, or straw, covered with a blanket or quilt. But when people sleep in feather-beds, they ought to air and beat them well in summer time once a week, and in winter once in a fortnight, and often change linen.

Q. 226.

Q. 226. What sort of bedding is proper for children?

A. Mattresses stuffed with straw, or moss well dried, which requires often to be changed.

Q. 227. Why ought they to lay on such beds?

A. Because it will contribute to the health, and promote the strength of children; and because feather-beds are more injurious to the health of children than to that of adults.

Q. 228. What is further to be observed with respect to sleep?

A. We ought not to lay down till we are tired, nor remain in bed after we wake in the morning.

Q. 229. Ought the head and breast be placed higher in bed than any other part of the body?

A. No; nor ought we to lay on our backs, but alternately on either side, in a somewhat bended position, taking care not to fold our arms round our heads.

Q. 230. Is it proper for children to sleep in the same bed with grown-up persons, or ought several children to lay together?

A. No. Such practices are very hurtful; for the breath and exhalations consist of noxious vapours: it is therefore adviseable for every child and every grown person to lay alone, in order to enjoy sound sleep.

Q. 231. What is to be done with beds in which sick people have lain?

A. They are for many days to be well aired and beat; but if the disease has been contagious, the bed ought to be burnt, or buried deep in the ground.

OBSERVATION.

An English army physician, Dr. Brocklesby, says, that a bed on which a person died of the quinsy, was the cause of the death of two others that slept in it after him. When travelling, one ought to be very careful and particular with respect to beds

XVI. *Of*

XVI. *Of the Habitations of Man.*

Q. 232. WHAT advantages ought our habitations and apartments to poffefs?

A. They ought to be very lightfome and airy.

Q. 233. When habitations are dark, rufty and damp, what effect do they produce on thofe that live in them?

A. People in fuch habitations are rendered unhealthy and weak, paralytic and fick; they grow ftupid, fimple, ill-natured, and miferable; and little children get pale in damp rooms; they fwell, become confumptive and die.

Q. 234. When may rooms be confidered as fufty and damp?

A. When they lay deep in the ground; when the walls and the floor are wet or damp, and when the furniture or other things grow mouldy.

Q. 235. How can fuch rooms be improved?

A. By the repeated and daily admiffion of frefh air into them; or, what is ftill better, by holes made in the two oppofite walls of the houfe, one near the floor, through which the external atmofphere conftantly paffes, and expulfes the foul air through the hole made near the cieling.

Q. 236. Ought rooms and chambers to be lofty and fpacious?

A. Yes; the more lofty and fpacious they are, the lefs liable will the air be to corruption.

Q. 237. How often ought they to be fwept and cleaned?

A. All inhabited rooms and chambers ought to be cleaned every day.

Q. 238. Why fo often?

A. Becaufe it is wholefome and good; and becaufe decent people like to live in clean apartments.

Q. 239. But is it good to fit in very warm rooms in winter time?

A. No. Very warm rooms are very unwholefome, and make people weak, fimple, ftupid, and fick.

Q. 240. Is it advisable to warm ourselves over charcoal, or to sit in rooms where it is burning.

A. No. Its vapours produce a great depression of spirits, and sometimes suffocate people.

OBSERVATION.

Those little stoves used by women in Germany and Holland to put their feet on are very dangerous.

Q. 241. Is it wholesome to dry clothes in rooms, or boil water in ovens, where the steam cannot ascend as in a chimney?

A. No. Damp vapours corrupt the air very much, and are therefore unwholesome and injurious to health.

Q. 242. If one be very much chilled in winter, may he immediately approach the fire, or a hot stove?

A. No; for chilblains are produced by exposure to heat after intense cold.

OBSERVATION.

Dipping the hands often in hot water, and sudden transitions from heat to cold, and from cold to heat, produce ulcers on the fingers, called in Germany " the worm."

Q. 243. When a limb, as an arm or leg, is frostbitten, what is best to be done?

A. In such a case if the patient enters a warm room, or approaches the fire, the loss of the arm or leg will be the consequence; the part affected should be kept in cold water, in which snow or ice was dissolved, till numbedness be removed, till life and sensation are restored.

OBSERVATION.

In cold winter days, if we travel or walk about in the country, it is necessary that we be particularly careful not to drink any brandy or other
spirituous

spirituous liquor, as it only tends to induce weariness and sleep, the more to be dreaded as it may last till death, through inanition, is produced.

Q. 244. What ought to be the state of rooms in which children live?

A. Their apartments ought to be lightsome and airy, and be kept orderly and clean; for in such rooms children will thrive surprisingly, and become healthy, strong, and cheerful.

XVII. *Of Schools.*

Q. 245. WHAT ought to be the site and state of a school-house?

A. It ought to be built in a free, open, and high situation; be dry, roomy, and in a good habitable condition.

Q. 246. What ought to be the state of school-rooms?

A. They ought to be lightsome, airy, large, high, and dry, having floors above the surface of the earth, not made of clay or stone, but of deal.

Q. 247. Are narrow, low, damp, dirty, dark rooms, which exclude the fresh air, unwholesome?

A. Yes; they are very unwholesome;—oppose the studies and intellectual improvement of children, and corrupt their morals.

OBSERVATION.

If men were sensible of these truths they would feel an irresistible impulse to unite, like so many bees in a hive, for the laudable purpose of promoting the general good—of erecting and establishing for the benefit of their children, healthy and spacious school-houses. They would be indemnified tenfold for their expences by the benign

nign influence such institutions would have in promoting the happiness of their offspring.

Q. 248. How ought school-rooms to be kept?

A. Orderly and clean, light and airy; taking care to open the doors and windows several times a day, in winter as well as in summer, for the admission of pure air, and not to keep too great fires in them.

XVIII. *Of Thunder and Lightning.*

Q. 249. HOW are people to conduct themselves in thunder-storms, when they are in the field?

A. They are not to run, trot, or gallop, or stand still, but keep on walking or riding quietly, slowly, and without fear.

OBSERVATION.

Here the school-master is to explain to the children the nature and causes of thunder and lightning, in order to prevent those fears and false impressions which are made upon the human mind, when children are suffered to form erroneous ideas of such phenomena.

Herds or flocks in thunder-storms ought not to be driven, hunted, or over-heated, or suffered to stand still, or assemble close together; they ought to be separated, and divided into small numbers; and people should take care not to come too near to them.

Q. 250. May one shelter himself in a tempest under a tree?

A. No; it is very dangerous. Trees, and vapours which encompass them, attract the lightning, and persons standing under them are in the utmost danger of their lives.

Q. 251. You are right, children, in observing that when thunder and lightning prevail, one should
not

not take shelter under trees; and the higher the tree the greater is the danger; but, what precautions are people to take when at home during a thunder tempest?

A. They are, when the tempest is still at a distance, to open the doors and windows of their rooms, chambers, and stables, in order to expel all vapours and fill them with fresh air. When the tempest draws nearer, the windows are to be shut and the doors left open, that fresh air may be admitted, avoiding carefully a free stream of air. They are further to keep at a proper distance from walls, chimneys, and ovens, and from all iron and metal, in particular from long iron rods or wires; remaining, as to any thing else, composed and without fear.

XIX. *Of over-heating Ourselves, and catching Cold.*

Q. 252. IF, through violent bodily exercise, labour, running, or dancing, we have over-heated ourselves, what ought we not to do?

A. 1. We ought not immediately to sit down or rest ourselves.

2. Drinking immediately after such violent exercise any thing cold, or even brandy or other spirituous liquor, is highly improper.

3. We ought not to expose our bare skin to the cold air.

4. We ought not to go into the cold bath: when thoroughly wet from rain it is proper to walk about.

5. We ought not to sit down on the ground, or on the grass; and we should be particularly careful not to fall asleep, otherwise ill-health, sickness, lameness, and consumption will be the fatal consequences.

OBSERVATION.

When people go home from their labour in the field, particularly in the evening, in cool, damp air,

air, they ought always firſt to put on their clothes, and not return in their ſhirts.

Q. 253. What elſe are we to attend to?

A. Thoſe that are over-heated are by very ſlow degrees to ſuffer themſelves to cool and enjoy reſt; and dry and clean ſhirts and clothes are to be ſubſtituted for thoſe that have been rendered humid by ſweat. When cool and compoſed we may gradually extinguiſh thirſt.

Q. 254. If people during work are very thirſty, may they not refreſh themſelves with ſome cold beverage?

A. Yes, they may; but they muſt not drink too much at once, nor leave off working and reſt themſelves, but continue their labour, elſe they will take cold and fall ſick.

Q. 255. What are thoſe to do who have caught cold from cold and damp wind and weather?

A. They are to drink a few cups of boiled water mixed with a fourth part of vinegar, put on warm clothes, and, by exerciſe, force the blood back to the ſkin. When the cold is violent, they are to bathe their feet in warm water, drink vinegar, and go to bed.

OBSERVATION.

It is very unwholeſome to drink ſpirituous liquors, or diaphoretics (medicines that induce perſpiration).

Q. 256. What are we to do if our feet or bodies be wet and cold?

A. We are to take off the wet ſtockings or clothes, leſt they ſhould cauſe a catarrh, the palſy, or rheumatiſm.

Q. 257. But what elſe ought to be done?

A. As ſoon as a perſon under ſuch circumſtances returns home he ought not only to take off the wet clothes, but waſh and dry his ſkin well, and put on warm clothes.

Q. 258. How do people by ſlow degrees get catarrhs, palſy, rheumatiſm, and other maladies?

A. By

A. By the obstruction of the perspiration, or rather transpiration, of the whole, or a part, of the body, occasioned by want of exercise, by wet or damp rooms or chambers, feather-beds, wet clothes, and exposure to cold air.

Q. 259. Point out to me, by way of elucidation, how a person may catch cold.

A. When a person, for instance, leans with his right or left arm against a damp wall, or, what is still worse, falls asleep in that position, or that the part is exposed to a stream of air, that part will be attacked by rheumatism or palsy, or catarrh will be produced.

Q. 260. How may catarrhs and rheumatisms be prevented?

A. They may be prevented by keeping the skin constantly cool, clean, and strong; by exposing it to pure air; by washing and bathing when the body is not kept too warm by unnecessary clothes, and by much exercise in the open air.

XX. *Of the Preservation of certain Parts of the Human Body.*

Q. 261. WHICH are the parts of the human body that man should take particular care to preserve in a good state of health?

A. The organs of his five senses.

Q. 262. By what means are the organs of the sight, the hearing, and smelling, preserved healthy, improved, and strengthened?

A. By free, pure air, and very frequent exercise in open air, rather than in confined places.

Q. 263. What is in general very hurtful to those three senses?

A. The unnecessary care of keeping the head warm by caps or other coverings, whereby the blood is drawn towards that part, evaporation obstructed, and

catarrhs

catarrhs and ulcers caused, the matter of which being absorbed, occasions blindness and deafness.

OBSERVATION.

The baneful consequences which arise from covering the head, or keeping it too warm, are ulcers, scabs, biles, and lice, which lay the foundation of evils to the human race greater than can be calculated.

Q. 264. How may the eyes be injured?
A. By dazzling, irregular, and transient lights; by objects brought too near the sight, or viewed sideways; by corrupted air, dust, smoke, damp vapours, the fat, sharp fumes of oil or candles; by the heat of ovens, and reading without sufficient light.

Q. 265. What hurts the hearing?
A. Strong, sharp, unexpected sounds or reports, corrupted air, feather-beds, dust, too much mucus in the nose, and pressure on the external ear, forcing it too near to the head.

OBSERVATION.

That the sense of hearing may be quick and distinct, the external ear should project sufficiently from the head and be moveable, but this is prevented by the close caps which young children wear.

Q. 266. How are the organs of smell injured?
A. By corrupted air; by strong and foul odours; by mucus in the nose, or snuff obstructing the nostrils, and obliging us to breathe through the mouth.

Q. 267. By what means is the organ of taste preserved?
A. By exercise; by the use of water, and bland aliment.

Q. 268. How may the organ of feeling be preserved?
A. By the exercise of the faculty of feeling; by the exercise of the body, and by cleanliness.

Q. 269. Are the common exercises of the senses sufficient to render them and reason perfect?

A. No. The senses require to be incessantly exercised that they may become perfect and capable of directing and upholding us amidst the wanderings of a disordered imagination, whose phantoms vanish before the torch of reason.

OBSERVATION.

Our sight and hearing, if not sufficiently improved, may deceive us during the night, or when the mental faculties are impaired by fear or prejudice: hence the origin of the absurd belief in spectres. But if our senses be rendered perfect; if we approach, and courageously endeavour to touch whatever imagination conjures up to our view, and that we explore whatever place a noise issues from, we shall soon be delivered from our delusion, and from the absurd belief in the existence of spectres, witches, and all such absurdities. Those who tell tales, and recount stories of spectres to children, with a view to frighten them, are highly reprehensible; and should be excluded from all share in the education of youth.

Q. 270. How can a good, intelligible pronunciation be obtained?

A. By keeping the mouth and the nose clean, the neck free and uncovered, and obliging children to accustom themselves to speak slowly, distinctly, and emphatically, and keep themselves erect.

Q. 271. Should we breathe through the mouth or the nose?

A. We should breathe through the nose, but not through the mouth; it is therefore necessary to keep the nose always clean by snuffing it, and to endeavour to breathe through the nose and keep the mouth shut during sleep.

Q. 272. Are there no other parts of the body which man should take particular care in preserving?

A. Yes;

A Yes; his teeth; for the teeth are not only neceſſary to aſſiſt us to pronounce diſtinctly, but for maſtication alſo; and on the proper maſtication of our food depends, in a great meaſure, digeſtion, and the nouriſhment, health, and proſperity of mankind.

Q. 273. How are the teeth injured?

A. By much fluid aliment; by coffee, tea, and other warm ſlops uſed inſtead of cold water; by corrupted air in apartments; by uncleanlineſs; by the uſe of tobacco; by bits of food, particularly meat, ſticking between them; by hot meats and liquors; by filling the mouth alternately with hot and cold things; by biting hard ſubſtances, and picking our teeth with knives, forks, pins, and needles; all which practices are highly injurious to them.

OBSERVATION.

Nobody ſhould put pins or needles in his mouth; they may eaſily be ſwallowed and cauſe death. In general it would be well to make as little uſe of pins, even in dreſſing, as poſſible.

Q. 274. By what means are the teeth preſerved ſound?

A. By the early habit of properly maſticating our food; by drinking cold water; by breathing pure air, and eating cold or tepid aliment, and drinking no warm liquors at all; by cleaning them after each meal either by drinking or gargling the mouth; and by refraining from picking of them: all this is neceſſary to keep the teeth ſound and beautiful.

Q. 275. By what means are the front teeth preſerved ſound?

A. By conſtant uſe, and the maſtication particularly of dry ſubſtances, as bread, &c.

OBSERVATION.

Children are not to cut with a knife the bread that has been handed to them, but to break it with the teeth and chew it.

Q. 276.

Q. 276. Should children alfo preferve their milk teeth?

A. By all means; for the lafting teeth, which are hid by them, are injured if the milk-teeth are not kept found by much chewing and maftication.

Q. 277. If the teeth be not kept found from childhood and are injured, can they be reftored to their original ftate?

A. No; that cannot be done; but through cleanlinefs, maftication, pure air, and cold water, injured teeth may be preferved from future injury.

Q. 278. What are the beft remedies to prevent tooth-ach?

A. Maftication, drinking of and gargling with cold water; pure air, cleanlinefs of the mouth, keeping the head cool, bathing the face after rifing in the morning and before going to bed in cold water.

Q. 279. Does the prefervation of the faliva deferve our particular notice?

A. Very much. The faliva is very neceffary in maftication and digeftion, and for that reafon the fmoking and chewing of tobacco, by which a great deal of the faliva is wafted, is a very bad cuftom, as is alfo the wetting of the thread when fpinning flax or hemp.

OBSERVATION.

The thread may be wetted with water which had been rendered clammy by beer, foap, ground linfeed, bran, thin dough, ftarch, kernels of quinces, bird-lime, or other things. And befides, the flax or hemp fhould be well beat before it is put on the diftaff, and well dufted, elfe, in fpinning, the duft or ligneous particles will be drawn by the breath into the lungs, and occafion coughing, ftuffing, and perhaps a confumption.

XXI. *Of the Beauty and Perfection of the Human Body.*

Q. 280. WHAT may be considered as one of the moſt appropriate qualities, and as a diſcriminative characteriſtic, of man?
A. His beauty.
Q. 281. What is the baſis of this beauty?
A. Health, and the perfect conformation of the body.

OBSERVATION.

" Health," ſays Bertuch (ſee Journal of Luxes and Faſhion), March 1793, page 189, " is the
" only and infallible ſource of beauty; all other
" modes of attaining it, ſuch as folly, impoſture,
" and ignorance have deviſed, may be compared
" to a plaſter, which ſoon falls off, leaving
" mournful traces of diſeaſe behind. The beau-
" tiful bloom of youth, the freſh colour, the ac-
" compliſhment of the whole bodily ſtructure,
" the free and eaſy play of the muſcles, the ful-
" neſs of the veins, the clear, delicately-ſpread,
" tranſparent ſkin, the glance of the eye ſo ex-
" preſſive of life and of the condition of the
" ſoul, cheerfulneſs extreme; all announce an
" inexpreſſible ſenſation of contentment and de-
" light, which diſpenſes health and happineſs
" both of ſoul and body, makes the huſband,
" the wife, the youth, the virgin, and the infant,
" happy, and beſtows on every member of ſociety
" charms and attractive powers which no art in
" the world can afford."

Q. 282. By what particular means may health be attained?
A. By free and eaſy exerciſe of the body during infancy.
Q. 283. What is beſides requiſite and neceſſary?
A. Free, pure air; waſhing and bathing; a light, eaſy dreſs; clear cold water for drinking; and ſimple good meals to nouriſh the body.

Q. 284.

Q. 284. By what means is the accomplifhment or perfection of the body to be attained?

A. By avoiding floth and inactivity till the twelfth year, after which plays and gymnaftic exercifes will bring the body to every degree of perfection of which it is fufceptible.

Q. 285. What is yet neceffary to facilitate the improvement of the body?

A. The inftruction of children in the various exercifes of the body which tend to render man healthy, ftrong, induftrious, and happy.

Q. 286. What pofture of the body ought we to recommend to children and to every one?

A. The erect pofture, whether we ftand or walk, keeping the breaft and head elevated; and on all occafions that will admit of it, an upright pofture is beft.

Q. 287. What, therefore, may be confidered as very hurtful?

A. Walking, ftanding, or fitting negligently, remaining bent or crooked, hanging down the head during infpiration, or while we fpeak or liften, and looking afkance.

Q. 288. Is it proper to accuftom children to make ufe on all occafions of the right hand only?

A. No; that is very wrong. Children are to be taught to make the fame ufe of the left hand as of the right.

Q. 289. What does moft diminifh beauty?

A. The habit which children fometimes contract of making wry faces and foolifh geftures.

Q. 290. Is the beauty of man all that depends on his accomplifhment or perfection?

A. No. Innocence and peace, reafon and virtue, the confcioufnefs of having done one's duty, and contributed toward the general good, in endeavouring to diffufe happinefs among mankind in this terreftrial abode, all fhew the accomplifhment, the beauty and dignity of man.

SECOND

SECOND DIVISION.

OF DISEASES.

XXII. *Of Diseases; Physicians, and Medicines.*

OBSERVATION.

IF people lived as they ought to do they would be exposed to very few internal complaints, perhaps to none at all; and the little ailments to which Nature under all circumstances is obnoxious, would be removed by those powers with which God has endowed her, for the preservation of the life and health of the human body, constructed with infinite wisdom and intelligence. But people, seduced by their passions and misguided by error, lead an irregular and dissolute life, and thus expose themselves to a train of melancholy diseases.

Q. 291. Tell me then, what ought those to do that are taken ill?

A. They ought to keep themselves tranquil and composed, and apply for the assistance of a physician.

Q. 292. What knowledge should a physician have who undertakes the cure of diseases?

A. He should have a thorough knowledge of the beautiful and complicated structure of the human body; know the proximate and remote causes of diseases, their nature and their mode of action on the human body; how the *vis medicatrix naturæ*, or sanative power of nature, operates; and how medicines, whose virtues he ought to be acquainted with, contribute to remove or cure diseases.

Q. 293.

Q. 293. Is the knowledge neceſſary for a phyſician eaſily attained, by reading a few books, or by converſation?

A. No. It is a very difficult matter to attain a thorough knowledge of the ſcience of phyſic, which we ſhould begin to ſtudy in our youth, and cultivate continually through life with great aſſiduity and pains.

Q. 294. To whom ſhould a patient apply for aſſiſtance?

A. Not to a quack, but a phyſician celebrated for his underſtanding, erudition, and rectitude of heart; who has received a regular education, and ſtudied methodically the very difficult art of knowing and curing diſeaſes.

Q. 295. What claſs of people do you call quacks?

A. All thoſe who are not acquainted with the ſtructure of the human body, and who have not methodically ſtudied the ſcience of curing diſeaſes; all thoſe who preſume to judge of the nature of a diſeaſe by the urine only; who arrogantly promiſe to cure every malady; and all thoſe are alſo claſſed among quacks who are not properly authoriſed to act in the capacity of phyſicians by ſome magiſtrate, univerſity, college of phyſicians, or ſome other reſpectable authority.

Q. 296. Is it poſſible to learn the nature of a diſeaſe from the urine?

A. No. The urine by itſelf cannot determine the nature of a malady. Thoſe, therefore, who ſet up as *water-doctors* are generally impoſtors; by whom many loſe not only their money, but their health and lives.

Q. 297. There are in every country preſumptuous, ignorant people, and in ſome parts Roman Catholic prieſts, executioners, ſhepherds, &c. who give themſelves an air of importance, have a great deal to ſay for themſelves, inſpect the urine, undertake to cure diſeaſes, and find every where employment and credit: —is it judicious to apply to ſuch people for aſſiſtance and remedies in caſe of ſickneſs?

A. No;

[71]

A. No; it is irrational; and people who apply to such quacks for help, prove that they are very ignorant and have been very badly instructed in their youth.

Q. 298. Can maladies originate in supernatural causes, such as witchcraft or sorcery?

A. No; it were nonsensical and foolish to believe it. Nature operates universally; and all diseases spring from natural causes.

Q. 299. What opinion may we form of travelling, advertising operators, that pretend to cure ruptures by section; and what are we to think of itinerant dentists and oculists?

A. They are mostly braggadocios, who have no other view than to defraud the credulous of their money.

Q. 300. Is it reasonable to buy medicines for man or beast of those medicine-hawkers who travel about the country?

A. No; for by the stuff which those vagabonds sell, life and health may be lost; their nostrums should not be given to any even of the brute creation.

Q. 301. Is it advisable to take domestic remedies?

A. No. In a hundred such there is hardly one that answers the purpose. The best, the only, and universal domestic remedies which the Almighty has given us are—fresh air and cold water.

Q. 302. What are we to observe respecting those universal, or secret medicines, for the cure, for instance, of canine madness, the ague, &c.?

A. Nothing favourable; they expose health and life to the utmost danger.

OBSERVATION.

The secret remedies against canine madness, and those which are usually resorted to as infallible, are good for nothing: they are not to be depended upon. The only certain means of preventing the fatal effects consequent on the bite of a mad dog (producing canine madness, shewn by a **strong abhorrence from water**), are, washing the
wound

wound as soon as possible with caustic lye, which destroys the surface of it; or, filling it and covering the edges of it with spanish-flies, which, by inducing copious suppuration, draw all the poison from the part affected.

Universal medicines (so called) are vainly exhibited for the cure of many, nay, even of all, diseases; but, in truth, there are no such medicines. The medicines so much recommended in newspapers, and the majority of English patent medicines, are good for nothing.

Q. 303. When people have received hurts on the exterior parts of the body, to whom are they to apply for assistance?

A. To a surgeon.

Q. 304. Is it very easy to attain a proper knowledge of surgery?

A. No. To become a good surgeon much study and labour are necessary.

Q. 305. Where ought those medicines to be bought that are prescribed by a physician or surgeon?

A. In the shops of apothecaries who are authorised to sell medicines, and who are noted for order and cleanliness, as well as for the ability with which they conduct business.

Q. 306. Is the art of an apothecary easily learnt?

A. No; it is very difficult; many years are required to become acquainted with all the medicines, to know their properties, and how to prepare them judiciously.

Q. 307. In what light are we to consider a physician in ordinary to a country?

A. He is the head, or chief physician, particularly authorised by the king, or the college of physicians, to take care of the health, and cure the diseases, of certain patients; and who, in cases of epidemic diseases, such as dysentery, putrid fevers, &c. is empowered to travel all over the country, for the purpose of investigating the causes of those diseases, and prescribing the most effectual remedies.

Obser-

OBSERVATION.

In some countries the chief business of physicians in ordinary is, to superintend and inspect all the apothecaries' shops in their respective provinces, to examine all the medicines, which, if good, they approve of; but they prosecute the apothecary, and confiscate his medicines, if they find them spurious.

Q. 308. At what period of a disease is it most proper to apply to a physician?
A. Immediately on the first attack.

Q. 309. What knowledge and information doth a physician require that he may be able to cure a disease?
A. He must know the nature and the cause of the disease: it is therefore indispensably necessary to acquaint him with all the incidental circumstances and symptoms of the disease, and to lay before him the whole state of the patient from the beginning of the malady, with the greatest exactness and accuracy; he must know the constitution, and the manner of living, of the patient, and likewise every circumstance which might have operated in producing the disease?

Q. 310. What is therefore proper?
A. That the physician see and speak to the patient himself, and investigate the nature and cause of the disease.

Q. 311. Suppose certain circumstances prevent this, what must then be done?
A. An exact and circumstantial statement of the case of the patient must be drawn by some intelligent person and sent to the doctor.

OBSERVATION.

In order to do this properly, every house-keeper, or, at least, every parish, in the country, in or near which there is no physician, ought to be in possession of certain rules, according to which such a statement may be drawn properly. I therefore apprize the public, that a book, much read in Germany, containing such rules, and much other useful

useful matter, is now translating and will soon be published.

Q. 312. What is required of a patient under the care of a physician?

A. That he take the medicines which the physician has prescribed, faithfully, regularly, in due time, and in the dose prescribed.

Q. 313. Is it to be expected that a serious indisposition should be cured by one prescription?

A. No. As well may we expect a large tree to be cut down by one stroke of an axe, as a disease of any consequence to be cured by the first prescribed physic.

Q. 314. If, then, the first prescribed medicine does not give relief, must the patient persevere in the use of it, or employ another doctor?

A. The patient must continue to take medicine till the disease be cured; but he must not go from one doctor to another.

Q. 315. Is it sufficient that the patient take the medicine prescribed, in order to obtain a cure?

A. No; it is not sufficient: he must observe a proper diet, without which medicines become of little use. Diseases are often cured by the healing powers of nature, assisted only by proper regimen.

XXIII. *Of the Conduct to be observed by Patients afflicted with Ardent Fevers.*

OBSERVATION.

THOSE diseases are denominated febrile which manifest themselves by cold or hot fits, and an unnatural alteration in the pulse, commonly accompanied with dislike to food, vomiting, weakness, anxiety, and pains all over the body, or in particular parts, and head-ach.

Q. 316.

Q. 316. A patient is a poor, helpless creature, oppressed by anxiety and pains;—how, then, ought he to be treated?

A. With the greatest tenderness, kindness, and affection; he ought to be attended and nursed with great and judicious care.

Q. 317. Is it proper to talk much to patients who suffer under grievous diseases, or to make great noise and confusion about them?

A. No. Patients ought as little as possible to be disturbed by talking; and every thing about them ought to be quiet.

Q. 318. Is it proper to admit visitors, or many persons, in the room where a patient lays?

A. No; because the air becomes corrupted by the breath and exhalations from so many visitors, who generally come through curiosity, and therefore ought not to be admitted.

Q. 319. What ought to be the state of the air in the rooms or chambers of the sick?

A. All patients, particularly those that labour under fever, ought to breathe fresh, pure, and dry air.

Q. 320. Is fresh air so necessary for a patient?

A. Yes. It is indispensably necessary for him; for it is most effectual in cooling and composing him, and diminishes anxiety.

Q. 321. What is further necessary?

A. That the room where the patient lays be aired by keeping the window open almost the whole day; that the windows and doors be thrown open occasionally, and that great care be taken not to expose the patient to gusts of air.

Q. 322. What kind of room is best adapted for a patient?

A. A dry, lofty and large room; not a low, narrow, damp, and musty room: it must be kept clean and orderly, all dust and nastiness expelled, and nothing suffered in it that can corrupt or infect the air.

Q. 323. Should the room of a patient be lightsome or dark?

A. It should not be very luminous, but rather darkish, as the light disturbs the repose of the patient.

Q. 324. What kind of bed doth the patient require?

A. An orderly and clean bed, not too warm, with covering not too heavy, bed not too soft, and clean linen. If straw be used instead of mattresses, it must be fresh and dry, and free from all offensive smell.

Q. 325. Is it good or bad for fever-patients to lay on feather-beds?

A. It is hurtful; for such beds augment the fever, and make it worse. Patients should lay on mattresses stuffed with horse-hair, or on straw, covered with a light quilt.

Q. 326. May two patients, or a patient and a person in good health, lay together in one bed?

A. No; every patient ought to have a bed to himself, and, if particular circumstances do not intervene, a room also: with respect to healthy persons, they ought not to sleep in the bed, or in the room, of a patient.

Q. 327. May the curtains of the bed be drawn in which a patient lays?

A. No; because it deprives him of the fresh air.

Q. 328. Ought not the bed of a patient to be shook and made daily?

A. Yes. A patient ought to be taken every day out of bed, at a time when he is not in a perspiration, that the bed may be made.

Q. 329. How ought a patient to be dressed?

A. His dress ought to be clean and comfortable.

Q. 330. Ought not the sheets of the bed, and the shirt or shift of the patient, to be changed?

A. Yes; they ought to be often changed; but the clean linen substituted ought to be well aired.

Q. 331. How ought the bed of a patient to be placed?

A. Not near a cold, damp wall, exposed to a stream of air; but in an open, free situation, that the patient may be approached and assisted on either side without inconvenience.

Q. 332. Is it proper to keep the heads of fever-patients, who are commonly very much affected with head-achs, warm?

A. No;

A. No; their heads are to be kept cool and uncovered, that the head-ach and delirium may not increase.

OBSERVATION.

By tying a bandage round the head the head-ach is often diminished.

Q. 333. What are patients to drink, particularly those who are afflicted with ardent fevers, which induce thirstiness?

A. Cold, pure water, which has for some time been exposed to the air, and thereby lost the greatest part of its chilliness. In fevers it ought to be mixed with vinegar or lemon-juice. A piece of toasted bread may also be added, being a good ingredient.

Q. 334. Is it good to warm or boil the water before it be given the patient?

A. No; it should neither be warmed nor boiled: for boiled water does not quench thirst nor compose the patient, nor is it at all good for such as are very thirsty.

Q. 335. Is it proper for patients to drink much tea?

A. No; it is commonly hurtful to them.

OBSERVATION.

The drinking of much warm tea is also very hurtful to women in child-bed: cold tea is preferable.

Q. 336. Do fever-patients like to drink cold water?

A. Yes. Cold water and fresh air are the best corroborants for fever-patients; they refresh, and diminish the anxiety and pains.

Q. 337. Must a fever-patient drink much water?

A. Yes: he ought to drink a great quantity; to quench his thirst it is necessary.

Q. 338. Doth cold water chill a patient afflicted with fever?

A. No; on the contrary, it makes him warm: a patient after drinking cold water falls often into a genial perspiration; and warm liquids frequently produce heat without any perspiration.

OBSERVATION.

In fluxes, pulmonic affections, and a few other diseases, warm drinks may perhaps agree better with the patient than cold.

Q. 339. May a patient labouring under fever drink beer, coffee, wine, brandy, or other spirituous liquors?

A. No; neither beer nor coffee; much less wine, brandy, or other spirituous liquors.

Q. 340. What regimen ought a patient to observe?

A. Patients afflicted with violent fever, or who labour under any other dangerous malady, lose all appetite, and therefore are not to be pressed to eat.

Q. 341. Why should not patients in a fever be pressed to eat?

A. Because they do not digest; and food remaining undigested in the stomach aggravates all diseases, particularly inflammatory fevers.

Q. 342. Is it proper to admit a patient afflicted with the first attack of fever to eat, if he has an appetite?

A. No; it is better for him to fast; for the eating of any thing readily increases the disease; fasting diminishes it; and there is no danger of starving.

Q. 343. What kind of nourishment had best be given a patient in fever, should he be desirous of any?

A. Butter-milk, sour milk, fresh, ripe, juicy fruits, raspberries, cherries, plums, grapes, baked or dried fruit, barley-water, or water-gruel mixed with vinegar or lemon-juice; and, in short, whatever can cool and refresh the patient.

OBSERVATION.

As fruit, whether fresh, dried, or made into jellies, is a most useful article, not only for the sick, but for general domestic use; and as fine fruit-trees are an ornament to a country, and a credit to the farmer; children ought, therefore, to be made
thoroughly

thoroughly fenfible of the great utility of planting good found fruit-trees, to be inoculated with the choiceft buds; and that it is their duty to promote the culture of fruit-trees with the utmoft affiduity.

In the next place, it is proper to fhew them how finful and fhameful it is to damage fruit-trees, bloffoms, or unripe fruit, or wafte ripe fruits by throwing fticks or ftones at them, or plucking them wantonly.

Near every burying-ground there ought to be a plantation of fruit-trees, propagated not from kernels only, but from fruits—from (for example) apples and pears, perfectly ripe, that have dropped or fallen from a found, fruitful tree;—fuch are to be planted like potatoes, lineally, in a plowed land, and be covered with thin or little earth. Two or three years after, the two ftrongeft of the four or fix faplings produced by each apple or pear are to be planted in an orchard or plantation, to ferve as ftocks, into which cyons may be engrafted.

The faplings propagated from the fruit itfelf will be a great deal more healthy, more fruitful, and durable, than thofe that are propagated from kernels only; and, if proper cyons be engrafted into them (perhaps without), the moft excellent fruits, in great abundance, may be expected.

Q. 344. What kinds of food are patients afflicted with fever to avoid?

A. Viands, broths, butter, eggs, heavy paftes, or bread not well fermented or baked, are not to be allowed to fuch patients.

Q. 345. When does their appetite return?

A. Not till the fever is cured, and reft and fleep reftored.

Q. 346. Should patients in general labouring under fever be kept warm or cool?

A. Such patients ought to be kept cool, avoiding all heat; and for that reafon great fires muft not be made in the room where the patient lays, for his fituation requires him to be kept more cool than warm.

Q. 347.

Q. 347. Is it good to sprinkle perfumes on the patient, or in his room?

A. Fresh air is better than all incense; but in malignant diseases it is very proper to correct the air by pouring vinegar upon red-hot iron repeatedly during the day.

OBSERVATION.

John Howard, that friend to mankind, who, in visiting and exploring prisons, hospitals, and lazarettos, sacrificed his life for the benefit of the human race, said, "The use of perfumes or in-
"cense is a clear demonstration of the want of
"cleanliness and fresh air."

Q. 348. Is it good to take any physic to promote perspiration?

A. No; in most cases it is dangerous; many fevers become by that means mortal. Such remedies or fluids that induce perspiration should therefore not be taken without the advice of a physician.

Q. 349. May a patient ill of a fever be bled?

A. It is in many fevers dangerous to bleed; and without the approbation of a physician no bleeding should take place in fevers.

Q. 350. But is it adviseable for people in good health to accustom themselves to be bled annually once or twice?

A. No. People that are in good health should never be bled; for by bleeding without necessity the blood is depraved, the body weakened, and health impaired.

OBSERVATION.

Bleeding pregnant women once or twice during their pregnancy is a very bad custom, hurtful both to mother and child.

Q. 351. Are emetics prescribed by a physician dangerous?

A. Emetics prescribed by a physician are not dangerous; they often do not weaken so much as purgatives.

OBSERVATION.

As many maladies, and particularly many fevers, originate in, or are connected with, a foulness of the stomach, emetics are often of very great service, as they expel all foulness from the stomach.

Q. 352. Should those who are ill of fever be permitted to remain long costive?
A. No. In fevers costiveness is very dangerous.

OBSERVATION.

For persons whose general health is good, and who are slightly indisposed, stewed, fresh, or dried fruit, particularly plumbs, are a good remedy against costiveness.

Q. 353. If a person be sick, and at the same time costive, by what means ought he to be relieved?
A. By a clyster.

Q. 354. Are clysters dangerous or doubtful remedies?
A. No; they are not.

Q. 355. What are we to observe with regard to the habit which some people have acquired of taking annually, at certain periods, purgatives?
A. It is a very bad custom; and medicines sold by pedlars and such vagabonds are commonly very pernicious.

Q. 356. Ought children in good health to be purged often?
A. No; it tends to nothing good; and in general the health of children should be preserved by proper attention, by nursing, and by much exercise in the open air, rather than by medicines.

Q. 357. Is it dangerous to blister in fevers, rheumatisms, gout, and many other diseases?
A. No; for Spanish-flies are not dangerous; they may be applied to little children, and render often much service.

Q. 358.

Q. 358. Is it good to make ufe of plafters and falves in cafes of wounds, contufions, or ulcers?

A. No; plafters and falves feldom do good in moft cafes they do more harm than good.

OBSERVATION.

In cafes of ulcers on the feet, or St. Anthony's fire in particular, plafters and falves are carefully to be avoided, as very bad, and productive often of obftinate fores.

Q. 359. What muft be done with wounds that are not very large and deep, where neither a great vein nor the bowels are hurt?

A. The wound muft be bandaged with a dry linen cloth, without being previoufly wafhed or cleanfed with brandy or water; for the blood, which is better than all plafters and falves, will perfectly cure the wound without any fuppuration.

Q. 360. What is beft to be done in cafes of contufion?

A. Linen cloths dipped in equal quantities of vinegar and water fhould be continually applied cold to the injured part: the pains will thus be abated, and the extravafated blood abforbed.

OBSERVATION.

Little ulcers may be dreffed with lint; or apply a linen bandage dipped in vinegar.

Q. 361. How are fcalded parts to be cured?

A. If (exactly as directed for contufions) linen cloths dipped in cold vinegar and water be applied from the beginning, and repeated every quarter of an hour, the burns will be cured better than by plafters and falves.

OBSERVATION.

Vinegar and water (equal parts) cures alfo fore nipples. Mothers may prevent forenefs of the nipples

nipples by washing them often in cold water before and after delivery.

XXIV. *Of Diseases which universally prevail; of Endemial, and of particular Maladies.*

Q. 362. IF diseases be very rife, and attack many, must the healthy take medicines, with a view of escaping from infection?

A. No; a healthy person should never take physic.

Q. 363. Should not people in such a case purge, take emetics, sweating potions, or be bled?

A. No; such weakening remedies would sooner beget than prevent infection.

Q. 364. Is it good to take corroborants for the stomach?

A. No; they are more hurtful than beneficial.

Q. 365. What should a person in good health do to escape general contagion?

A. He should be very temperate in eating and drinking, observe cleanliness, take a great deal of exercise, and be careful not to over-heat himself or to catch cold.

OBSERVATION.

In times of scarcity putrid fevers and contagious diseases, which sometimes depopulate whole provinces, are caused by eating bad bread, and by unwholesome food in general.

Q. 366. Is no other precaution necessary?

A. Yes; and as diseases that generally prevail are often contagious, we should not expose ourselves to danger by visiting patients, nurses, or hospitals.

Q. 367. When certain diseases, for instance the ague, are endemial, and that stagnant waters or morasses in the neighbourhood are the causes of such fevers, what should the inhabitants do?

A. They

A. They ought to drain the waters and dry the moraſſes and the fever will ceaſe; for with the cauſe the effect naturally ceaſes.

Q. 368. If mechanics or artiſts be often attacked by diſeaſes peculiar to them, a ſtone-maſon, for inſtance, with conſumption, painters with cholic, what ought they to do?

A. They ought, as ſenſible men, who wiſh to be healthy and live long, to inveſtigate the true cauſe of their frequent diſeaſe, and ſtrive to find out how they can diminiſh or avoid it.

OBSERVATION.

Thoſe who lead a ſedentary life, females, mechanics, artiſts, the ſtudious, ought, from their infancy till the complete ſhedding of the teeth in the twelfth year, to be exhorted or obliged to take a great deal of bodily exerciſe in the open air, in order that future inactivity and confinement may not injure their health and happineſs too much.

XXV. *Of Contagious Diſeaſes.*

Q. 369. WHICH diſeaſes are peculiarly contagious?

A. Putrid fevers, ſpotted fevers, dyſentery, the yellow and ſcarlet fever, ſmallpox, and meaſels. The plague, the worſt of all diſeaſes, is very infectious.

Q. 370. How do they communicate infection?

A. By contact, or through the medium of the atmoſphere, impregnated with putrid miaſms, ariſing from the perſpiration of patients labouring under any of thoſe diſeaſes.

Q. 371. What is particularly to be obſerved with reſpect to alleviating the ſymptoms which obtain in contagious diſeaſes?

A. The

A. The air, as well in the room as in the house where the patient lays, ought to be preserved continually pure and fresh, by keeping one window always, and the windows and doors occasionally, open. In short, one cannot be too assiduous in procuring constant fresh air.

Q. 372. What is further to be observed?

A. The greatest cleanliness ought to be observed with regard to the patient, the bed, the room, and attendants, observing not to keep the room too warm.

Q. 373. What else should be done to guard against infection?

A. Previous to visiting a patient we should take some nourishment;—we should, however, avoid eating any thing in the apartments of the sick; guard ourselves against infection by good cheer and fortitude, and, as far as we can, administer relief and comfort.

Q. 374. What duties do those who are intrusted with the care of patients owe to their fellow-creatures?

A. They ought, in order to prevent the infection from spreading, to keep by themselves, avoid all unnecessary intercourse with other people, and not enter any school or church; and the children and domestics of patients should be placed under the same restraint.

OBSERVATION.

To schools contagious diseases are often communicated by children, and so spread to distant parts.

Q. 375. May many persons be admitted into the room of a patient who is infected with a contagious disease?

A. None but those that are intrusted with the care of the patient; and all curious visitors should be refused admittance without any ceremony.

Q. 376. Why is it a duty incumbent on the healthy to avoid approaching an infected person when there

there is no preffing neceffity that impels us to expofe ourfelves to contagion?

A. Becaufe felf prefervation, and what we owe to our families and fellow-creatures, directs us not to endanger our own health, and efpecially not to endanger the health of our fellow-creatures.

Q. 377. If an infected perfon dies, what is then to be done?

A. The corpfe muft not be expofed to public view, but buried as foon as poffible, avoiding funeral pomp, and admitting but few to attend the bier.

Q. 378. Is not the itch a contagious difeafe?

A. Yes; it is a moft abominable diftemper, which is communicated very readily by contact with an infected perfon.

Q. 379. What muft be done to efcape this difeafe?

A. We muft avoid the company of infected perfons.

OBSERVATION.

Children who have the itch or fcurfy heads fhould not be admitted into fchools, that other children may not be infected. If fchool-mafters, as it is their duty, would take the trouble of examining the hands of their pupils, and would command them to be wafhed daily before coming to fchool, children fo infected would foon be found out.

Q. 380. Is it dangerous in cafes of itch, fcurf, or leprofy, to ufe fulphur ointment?

A. Yes; it is very dangerous; and may occafion lofs of health, blindnefs, and deafnefs.

XXVI. *Of the Small-pox.*

Q. 381. F ROM what can the degree of danger in fmall-pox be conjectured?

A. Chiefly

A. Chiefly from their number. If the pustules be few there is little danger; but where they are many, and confluent, the danger is great.

Q. 382. What is therefore lucky?

A. To have but few pustules.

Q. 383. At what period of the disease may we apprehend danger?

A. Not at the beginning when the pustules come forth, but towards the end, when they suppurate and dry, and when the matter is absorbed into the system and excites a secondary fever.

Q. 384. When a child has symptoms of being infected with this disease, is it proper to have recourse to wine, brandy, warm rooms, and feather-beds, to forward the eruption?

A. No; it would be acting very injudiciously; for by such means we would increase the number of pustules, and consequently the danger.

Q. 385. What is then to be done?

A. The cure must be left to nature, observing only, during the period of the eruptive fever, which lasts two, three, or four days, to keep the patient cool and in fresh air, allowing him but little nourishment, and cold water only for drink.

Q. 386. When at last the pustules are forced out by the fever, what must be done in the course of the disease, and during the concoction of the matter?

A. We should keep the patient in a situation where the air is pure and dry; give for drink cold water, and enjoin temperance and moderation in eating and drinking.

Q. 387. Is it good to lay in bed in the day-time at the period of the eruptive fever, before the eruption of the small-pox, and during the whole course of the disease?

A. No; it is not good in the day-time: the patient, if possible, should keep out of bed, and at night lay in a bed that is not too warm nor fusty; feather-beds are therefore very hurtful to this class of patients.

Q. 388. When the eye-lids are ulcerated and clofed, is it right to force them open, and apply to, or blow into, them fpices, or other hot things?

A. No; the eye-lids muft not be forced open, or meddled with, nor ought inflammatory things, which induce blindnefs, to be applied to them; but when at laft they open of themfelves care muft be taken that they be not irritated by too much light in the room, which fhould be kept darkfome, both before and after they open. Particular attention is alfo to be paid to keeping the air in the room pure and cool.

Q. 389. Is great mortality occafioned by the fmall-pox?

A. Yes; in general out of ten patients labouring under the natural fmall-pox, one dies.

ADDRESS TO CHILDREN.

Children, the natural fmall-pox is a bad diftemper —as bad as the plague! But an omnifcient Being has, in his goodnefs, enabled man to find out a remedy for the alleviation of the great miferies occafioned by it. He has led us to the important difcovery of inoculation, which deftroys in a great degree the virulence of this baneful difeafe, which at laft, we may hope, will be entirely eradicated.

When children are inoculated they have only a few puftules of the beft kind; they are feldom confined to bed; feldom lofe their health; and of a hundred inoculated hardly one dies; whereas one out of ten of thofe afflicted with the natural fmall-pox generally dies.

Q. 390. Do you wifh to be made acquainted with the procefs of inoculation?

A. Yes; if you will be fo kind as to explain it.

INSTRUCTIONS HOW TO INOCULATE.

In order to inoculate a child in a good ftate of health, a needle is dipped in a little frefh, thin small-pox-matter of a child that is infected with a good, distinct, and true small-pox, with few pustules. With this needle an incision is made of the breadth of a straw under the scarf skin of both arms above the elbow, without drawing any blood, so that the matter shall be lodged under the upper skin; and this is called inoculation for the small-pox.

The effect produced, and the conduct to be observed by the patient, I shall point out, and is as follows: Having the great advantage of knowing to a certainty that the person inoculated must have the small-pox within ten or fourteen days, the strictest regularity and temperance with regard to diet is to be enjoined.

The fourth, fifth, or sixth day the incisions become inflamed, red, thick, and hard; and from this time till the complete restoration of the patient to perfect health, the incisions, which are often much inflamed, and from which a great deal of matter oozes, ought to be repeatedly washed every day with cold water.

The seventh, eighth, or ninth day after the inoculation the patient feels pains under the arms, and is attacked by head-achs, fever, and sometimes vomits.

This fever lasts two, three, or four days, during which period the patient should not remain in bed, but, though it may be very inconvenient in the beginning, walk, or be carried, about where here is fresh, pure, cool air, which is absolutely necessary.

In free and cool air fever and head-ach vanish; and if the forehead and arms be frequently washed in cold water, almost all illness will go off.

The second, third, and fourth day of the fever, or the tenth, eleventh, or twelfth day after inoculation, sometimes later, the small-pox come forth of their own accord. they ought not to be forced to make their appearance.

In most cases there are very few pustules, which, being very good, the disease is soon at an end.

The pustules in this case contain very little matter, and dry soon; and it is only necessary to keep the patient regular and in fresh air, to prevent the disease from becoming dangerous.

Q. 391. But tell me, my dear children, may inoculation be performed in a place that is yet free from the contagion of the small-pox?

A. No; because the small-pox is a contagious disease, and by inoculation might be carried to distant parts, and, what would be a great misfortune, occasion the death of many children that otherwise might have escaped infection.

Q. 392. But may inoculation be performed in places which are already infected?

A. No; even that is wrong; for the inoculated may infect one single person, and be the accidental cause of his death.

Q. 393. Where, then, should children be inoculated?

A. In houses set apart for inoculation, that are erected for that purpose at a proper distance from other habitations, and where there is no danger of infecting other people.

ADDRESS TO CHILDREN.

You are right, children; inoculation should only take place in houses devoted to that purpose; whoever acts otherwise commits a crime against society.

Q. 394. Can a person be infected twice by the small-pox?

A. No; the true small-pox cannot infect the same person more than once: all stories of getting the infection twice are erroneous.

XXVII. *Of the Measles.*

Q. 395. ARE the measles a bad distemper?
A. Yes; they take away the lives of many; and even

even after they go off leave behind complaints which too often prove fatal.

Q. 396. What may particularly be observed with regard to this disease, whose action is so inimical to the breast or lungs?

A. Patients afflicted with it must be kept a little warmer than is necessary in cases of small-pox, but not too warm; they ought to breathe pure air, and drink elder-flower tea; and great care is to be taken that they do not expose themselves to cold air or sudden gusts of wind.

Q. 397. When this disease goes off, what are we to do for the patient, that, from the injuries done to his constitution, he may not fall a victim to consumption?

A. The patient for some time must guard against the open air, and put on warm cloathing.

OBSERVATION.

This necessary precaution ought also to be taken in cases of yellow and scarlet fevers; for as in these diseases, as well as in the measles, the whole scarf skin scales off, it is very easy to catch cold, the consequence of which would be dropsy, consumption, or other bad and fatal complaints.

XXVIII. *On the entire Extirpation of the Small-pox and Measles.*

ADDRESS TO CHILDREN.

DEAR children, the small-pox is a kind of plague, nay, worse than a plague, causing still more misery. In Berlin, 1077 persons fell victims to this disease in 1786; in the duchy of Mecklenburgh Schwerin, 2695 in 1791: and in Upper Silesia, 5584 in the space of three years. From the year 1650 till 1750, being a century, 152,461 persons fell sacrifices to this baneful disease in London; and in Sweden, 95,101 lost their

their lives by the small-pox and measles in the space of eleven years.

One thousand years ago the small-pox was not known in Europe. It was transmitted to us from the burning regions of Africa, where the plague is endemic; and, owing to our ignorance and inattention, has established itself among us. Every one, almost without exception, contracts this distemper, either through his own fault in exposing himself imprudently to the infection, or by being exposed by others; and one patient out of ten is generally cut off.

If we now but for a moment consider the numbers that are swept away by this disease—the thousands and hundred thousands of the human race that perish through its baneful influence, we must confess it is one of the greatest and most horrid plagues that human kind has to encounter.

Q. 398. But perhaps this African plague is an evil necessary for the human race?

A. No; it is not a necessary evil; else it would have prevailed among us from time immemorial; whereas, one thousand years ago every one enjoyed a good state of health, without having had the small-pox.

Q. 399. You are right, children, the small-pox is not natural to the human race, or conducive to health. Tell me, then, how is this disease communicated?

A. By infection only.

Q. 400. But cannot people contract it by an irregular method of living;—by irregularity in eating and drinking, and exposure to an inclement sky?

A. No. It can only be propagated by infection floating in the atmosphere, or by inoculation.

Q. 401. If therefore a person takes great care not to be infected, what follows?

A. That such a person escapes the disease.

Q. 402. And if every one living were to take the same precautions to avoid infection, what would be the consequence?

A. That

A. That no one would ever be afflicted with the small-pox.

Q. 403. And if no one were to be afflicted with the small-pox, no one therefore could communicate it to another; what then would be the natural consequence?

A. That the small-pox would be completely exterminated.

ADDRESS TO CHILDREN.

Children, listen to me. The plague is just like the small-pox, a disease which cannot originate itself, but must be communicated by contagion. In former centuries the plague was very common, and generally known. It raged in Germany in the years 1712 and 1713; and in London in 1665 and 1666. To this wide-wasting pestilence one-third of mankind have often fallen sacrifices. But people at last grew wiser. The infected were separated from the healthy; all communications with towns and places, where the plague raged, was cut off, and every possible care taken to prevent the contagion from spreading; so that at last this scourge to human-kind was radically extirpated.

The small-pox is as shocking and dreadful in its effects as the plague, and might as easily be extirpated.

Q. 404. What do you conclude from this?

A. That it is the duty of man to extirpate the small-pox, and that without any loss of time.

ADDRESS TO CHILDREN.

You are right, children, in saying that it is the duty of man to extirpate the small-pox, and to take immediately the most effectual measures for obtaining so desirable an end.

The best regulations have been made with regard to preventing or curing the diseases to which the brute creation is obnoxious. It would therefore be a great and just reflection upon mankind if they

they neglected using every possible means for exterminating the small pox,—a horrid disease, which robs the earth of the tenth part of its inhabitants, and spreads misery and devastation among the infant poor, whom it afflicts with excruciating pains and torments.

It is then a consolation to observe that this disease can, and therefore ought to be extirpated in the following manner.

But it is proper first to inform you that the matter of the small-pox, whether fluid or dry, contains the infectious poison, which is capable of propagating the disease; that the air which we breathe is not contagious, and perhaps only becomes so when saturated with a great quantity of putrid exhalations from patients, and that therefore it behoves us to keep the air fresh and pure.

XXIX. *Instructions how to Exterminate the Small-pox by easy Means, in which every Individual is bound to concur.*

1. IN the environs of every city and town, a house, built agreeable to a particular plan, should be appropriated for the reception of patients infected with the small-pox; and there should be an adjoining building of lesser size.

OBSERVATION.

The expences of such an undertaking will be inconsiderable. At Berlin only, in a single year, 1786, one thousand seventy-seven persons fell miserable victims to the small-pox. What, then, is the expense of an hospital, when compared with the loss to the community of so many of our fellow-creatures?—Nothing!

2. All inhabitants of adjacent towns and villages, even travellers, ought to contribute towards the support

port of this hospital, as all are interested in its establishment.

3. All those who live within the district where the hospital is built, even the children in the schools, should be provided with a complete description, elucidated with prints, of the various diagnostic symptoms of the real small-pox, and the duty, necessity, and utility of delivering over infected persons and children to that hospital, should be pointed out and inculcated.

4. As soon as any person, young or old, poor or rich, inhabitant or stranger, has received the contagion, such person should immediately, and without any loss of time, be sent to the hospital, and thus be separated for a little time from that society to which he had become dangerous. This is unavoidably necessary, and a duty we owe to the community at large. But as soon as hospitals for the small-pox are properly established, this disease will become far less frequent, and will only take place with a few; for every body, from a dread of being sent to the hospital, will do all he can to keep himself and family free from the infection.

5. The names, both christian and surname, and the places of abode, of all infected persons, should be accurately pointed out and published in several newspapers, and information thus given that certain persons, properly described in the advertisement, have been sent to the small-pox hospital (specifying the county in which such hospital is situated): an inquiry should then be made respecting the source of the infection thus communicated, and all persons suspected taken up and sent to the hospital.

6. When the patient arrives at the hospital, he is first introduced into the adjoining building, there stripped of all his clothes and linen, and provided with clean and wholesome apparel.

7. The clothes he has taken off are cleaned, washed, fumigated, and exposed to fresh air.

8. The patient in the hospital is placed under the care of nurses, whose duty it is carefully to attend him,

him, and provide him with the best and cleanest food. He has besides the assistance of the ablest physicians and surgeons: in short, the tenderest care is taken of him.

9. Whoever is to be inoculated should be sent to the hospital, for inoculation should not be permitted any where else.

10. None but such as have had the small-pox ought to be admitted into the hospital as visitors.

11. Parents may attend in the hospital and nurse their own children, and friends their friends, provided they have had the small-pox; if not, they must suffer themselves to be inoculated, and submit to the order of the house.

12. The nurses appointed to attend in the hospital, and even parents that nurse their children, are to make very few excursions from the hospital; none secretly or clandestinely; but, if they must go out, they should always first take off their infected clothes, wash themselves in the baths of the adjoining building all over, and particularly the hair, and then put on clean, uninfected clothes; and this rule ought also to be observed by every body that enters the house.

13. The physician and surgeon ought to change their clothes and linen in the adjoining building, before they enter the hospital; and before they depart should wash at least their faces and hands, and change their clothes.

14. Forty or sixty days after the complete extirpation of this horrid plague, the patient, after he has been well cleansed, washed, and bathed from top to toe, and after having put on clean clothes and linen, is restored to society, which circumstance should be published in the newspapers.

15. Eight days after a patient is discharged in good health from the hospital, he is to be brought to the temple of God, where *Te Deum* is to be sung by the whole enraptured congregation.

ADDRESS TO CHILDREN.

And thus, dear children, in so easy a manner, and by so excellent an institution, the most horrid

and

and disgusting disease—a disease which consigns to misery and death a great portion of mankind—may be thoroughly extirpated. European nations will at last become sensible of this truth, and see the absolute necessity of exterminating a plague, which must vanish from among them if they only will it.

If a few hospitals, such as I have described, were erected, many towns and villages would be freed from this disease; and distant nations would follow the laudable example of erecting public edifices to restrain and diminish the infection of the small-pox, and banish it from villages, towns, and provinces.—And, dear children, rejoice with me in the glorious prospect of their success.

In ten or twenty years the plague called the small-pox, which torments and sweeps annually from the earth the tenth part of the human species, will, if the plan proposed be adopted, be entirely exterminated.

Q. 405. But tell me, children, could not the small-pox be exterminated in a shorter period than ten years?

A. O yes; it could be extirpated in a much shorter time, if man (and it is his duty) would immediately and seriously begin to make the necessary arrangements for it, and erect hospitals.

OBSERVATION.

The extermination of the small-pox has actually taken place in Louisiana and Chili, and other countries. In North America, in Rhode Island, which is very populous, fourteen miles long and seven broad, enjoying a great commerce, inoculation is prohibited; but every person infected by the small-pox is immediately removed to a small island at a short distance, called *Coasters' Harbour*, and is compelled to stay there till all danger of infection has ceased.

Dr. Waterhouse says of these regulations, " The " terror which this contagion has spread among

"the inhabitants induces them cheerfully to sub-
"mit to them; and should a stranger suppose
"that they cannot be observed so scrupulously
"without compulsion, he will find himself mis-
"taken. The unanimous voice of the people,
"and the vigilance of the magistrates, insure the
"desired effect; so that the regulations we allude
"to seem to be more the custom of the country
"than a restraint imposed by the law."

Even a certain people that are held in universal detestation on account of their uncleanliness, ignorance, and barbarity, the *Hottentots*, when the small-pox first began to exert its baneful influence amongst them, separated the sick from the healthy by ramparts, at which sentinels were placed, and thus the spreading of the contagion was prevented.—And we Europeans, with all our civilization, reason, and sciences, are we to yield the palm of humanity to Hottentots?—Forbid it, Heaven!

The measles also, in all probability, first made their appearance in Africa, whence this disease was brought over to us, a thousand years ago, with the small-pox. Like the plague and the small-pox, it is not a necessary evil: it is propagated only by infection; may be considered as a very bad disease, which is often fatal. In 1751, five hundred and twenty-three persons died of it in Berlin, in the space of eighteen weeks.

Q. 406. Would it not be possible to extirpate the measles as well as the small-pox?

A. Yes; and in the same manner, and by the same regulations, as those pointed out for the extirpation of the small-pox; and it is our bounden duty to attempt it.

OBSERVATION.

If the scarlet fever, dry or hooping cough, and the itch also, were only propagated by infection, they might be exterminated with equal success.

XXX. *Of the Bloody-Flux, or Dysentery.*

Q. 407. At what season doth the bloody-flux commonly appear?

A. In the summer, but mostly in the autumn.

Q. 408. Is the bloody-flux a bad and dangerous disease?

A. Yes; it is a very malignant disease, exposing the patient to great danger if he be improperly treated.

Q. 409. Is the bloody-flux the consequence of eating fruit?

A. No; ripe, sweet, juicy fruits, particularly grapes, rather prevent, than produce, this disease.

Q. 410. What precautions ought to be taken to avoid infection?

A. People should be very careful in avoiding cold, especially observing to keep the belly warm; eating much ripe fruits, particularly grapes, and good meats.

Q. 411. What is further to be observed?

A. The new corn, before it is made into bread, ought to be perfectly ripe and dry; and the bread made of it ought to be thoroughly baked, and not be eaten when warm or too new. New, unripe potatoes are dangerous also, and all vegetables which are often blighted or injured by insects ought to be well washed and cleaned before they are boiled.

Q. 412. The stomach and bowels of patients labouring under dysentery are filled with bitter, acrid, and putrid matter:—Is it proper to endeavour to stop the progress of the disease by confining this matter, the cause of the disease, in the stomach and bowels?

A. No. The stopping of the bloody-flux would endanger life; but the body ought to be cleansed by emetics and purges immediately at the beginning of the disease.

Q. 413. What ought therefore to be avoided?

A. The stopping of the flux by the fat of mutton, sweet-oil, spices, pepper, Venice treacle, wine, or spirituous liquors, which endanger life.

Q. 414. What is further to be observed, as the bloody-flux is often infectious?

A. The

A. The greatest cleanliness; filling the patient's chamber with fresh air, and taking great care that any excrements, as soon as voided, be carried out of the room, and buried under much earth.

Q. 415. Is it necessary to consult a physician in case of dysentery?

A. A physician ought to be consulted in every disease, particularly in dysentery, which is extremely dangerous.

XXXI. *Of Treatment, after Diseases are removed.*

Q. 416. WHAT ought to be observed after heavy diseases are removed?

A. Regularity and temperance in eating and drinking, taking only light nourishing food, and observing not to expose ourselves too soon to the weather.

Q. 417. And may a person just restored to health set to work immediately?

A. No; a person just risen from the bed of sickness ought first completely to recruit his natural strength and vigour before he begins to work again.

XXXII. *Of Public Institutions for the Sick.*

OBSERVATION.

CHILDREN, if we consider the numberless unhappy and miserable wretches that are scattered over the surface of the earth, afflicted with diseases and poverty, unable to promote their own, or the happiness of their fellow-creatures, depending on the bounty and labour of others for their support, causing embarrassment, anxiety, and trouble to society, to whom they are unable to make any compensation, we must acknowledge that diseases are evils of the greatest magnitude, afflict,

afflict, not only particular individuals but the community at large, and imbittering the cup of life.

Q. 418. By what means can people avoid those evils?

A. By observing the two following rules:

1. That all persons, particularly children, be instructed respecting the nature of the human body, and the means of preserving health, with a view of extending life beyond the usual period, and guarding ourselves as much as possible against disease and death.

2. That all patients receive the best attendance and nursing, and all possible assistance and help from physicians and surgeons.

Q. 419. Do all patients receive such necessary attendance and assistance?

A. No; they are too often neglected.

Q. 420. What reasons can be assigned for the greater number of patients not receiving the necessary assistance and attendance?

A. The ignorance, the poverty, and the misery of so many people; their wretched and unwholesome habitations; want of constant fresh air; uncleanliness; bad, loathsome beds; and the indigence of so many people, which prevents them from calling in a physician or surgeon, or procuring medicines.

ADDRESS TO CHILDREN.

You are right, dearest children; diseases not only become through those circumstances dangerous and mortal, and sources of the greatest misery to patients and their families who live by their industry only, but they also become at last contagious, and spread their baneful influence far and wide over the human race.

It is true that people may be delivered from their ignorance by proper instructions regarding the attendance and nursing of patients, and thereby be rendered capable of serving their fellow-creatures; yet all patients cannot help themselves;

and there will be still many poor sufferers left, who in vain will demand or seek for assistance.

Q. 421. What, therefore, should we do for the preservation of the lives and health of our poor fellow-creatures?

A. We ought to erect every where hospitals, or appropriate houses for the same purpose; and take care that all poor, indigent, diseased persons find in those habitations the best accommodations; or that every assistance be administered to them *gratis* * in their own houses, which ought to be kept clean. Patients in either case should have the assistance *gratis* of such physicians and surgeons as are generally esteemed for their rectitude, humanity, and abilities.

Q. 422. Why should man establish such institutions?

A. Because it is his duty.

ADDRESS.

Yes, dear friends, it is your bounden duty to erect hospitals for the reception of your poor, sick, helpless, unfortunate brethren—for we are all children of the All-Bountiful Heavenly Father, who ordained mutual love and charity among mankind, and beholds the mansions of the sick and unfortunate as temples erected to Himself.

Q. 423. What good may we expect from such institutions?

A. That human misery will be diminished, and the lot of mankind meliorated.

Dr. C. L. Lenz has made the extirpation of the small-pox, the measles, and all contagious maladies, the chief object of his life, his researches, and his studies; and those works of his which treat of these weighty concerns, so very important to the human race, and which are intended to be published, deserve

* *Res sacra est miser.*
  Misery is sacred.

the greatest attention. As soon as completed, I shall presume to offer the public a correct translation of them, for which I have made the necessary preparatory arrangements.

THE TRANSLATOR.

OBSERVATION.

It would be highly meritorious in physicians to instruct the school-masters of their respective districts in the contents of this Catechism of Health, which is also translated into most of the European languages, and universally adopted in schools as a book of instruction.

ORDER

ORDER OF THE HUMAN TEETH.

J. Hunter's Natural History of the Human Teeth, London 1771.

Sommering's Doctrine of Bones, P. XVIII. and page 192—223.

A. Milk Teeth.

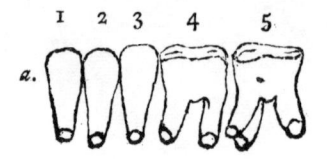

B. Lasting Teeth.

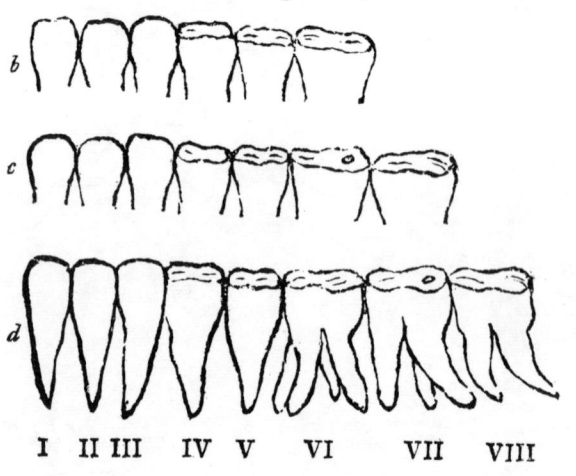

The number and strength of the teeth depend on the nourishment of the body by solid food, and on the health and strength of the human body. The most remarkable changes, respecting the number, as well as the strength, of the teeth, take place during infancy, and from the period of youth till the age of maturity; and our education ought to accord with this divine ordination of nature.

The first row of teeth *(a)* is that of a child.
The second *(b)* that of a boy and girl.
The third *(c)* that of a youth and virgin.
The fourth *(d)* that of a man and woman.

I and 1, II and 2, are two cutting-teeth; III and 3, are corner or eye-teeth, and IV and 4, V and 5, VI, VII, VIII, are jaw-teeth, *molares*; of which the child has on each side of each jaw two, boys and girls three, youths and virgins four, and men and women five.

THE

THE ORDER AND THE PERIODS OF HUMAN LIFE.

I. FOETUS

(generated by healthy Parents).

II. SUCKLING.

III. INFANT.

Cutting of the *Milk Teeth* in both Jaws.

Month	M. T.	1	2	3	4	5
8	2	2	0	0	0	0
10	4	4	0	0	0	0
12	8	4	4	0	0	0
16	12	4	4	0	4	0
20	16	4	4	4	4	0
24	20	4	4	4	4	4

IV. CHILD.

Perfect *Milk Teeth* in both Jaws.

Years	M. T.	1	2	3	4	5
3 till 7	20	4	4	4	4	4

V. Disciple.

Shedding of the *Milk Teeth* in both Jaws.

Year	M. T.	1	2	3	4	5
7	18	2	4	4	4	4
8	14	0	2	4	4	4
9	10	0	0	4	2	4
10	6	0	0	4	0	2
11	2	0	0	2	0	0
12	0	0	0	0	0	0

Cutting of the *Lasting Teeth* in both Jaws.

Year	L. T.	I	II	III	IV	V	VI
7	4	0	0	0	0	0	4
8	8	4	0	0	0	0	4
9	12	4	4	0	0	0	4
10	16	4	4	0	4	0	4
11	20	4	4	0	4	4	4
12	24	4	4	4	4	4	4

Lasting Teeth in both Jaws.

Years	L.T.	I	II	III	IV	V	VI	VII	VIII	
12 till 16 or 18	24	4	4	4	4	4	4	0	0	VI Boy and Girl
16 or 18 till 20 or 24	28	4	4	4	4	4	4	4	0	VII Youth and Virgin
20 or 24 till senile age	32	4	4	4	4	4	4	4	0	VIII Man and Woman.

IX. Senile Age.

X. Close of Life.

STATE OF PERFECT HEALTH.

THE health and happiness of mankind will be brought to a state of perfection when marriage is ordained to take place only between healthy persons, descended from healthy parents; for the first and most important requisite to a state of perfect health to endure till senile age is, an origin from healthy parents. *

The next chief requisite to a perfect and lasting state of health, is, that the suckling and infant experience in the highest degree possible the love and care of the mother; that children, without any distinction as to sex, be clothed in the garment represented in the frontispiece; live in society with other children in the open air, and so improve their bodies and their minds.

And it is also of great importance that the body, after the twelfth year, or after the shedding of the teeth, be strengthened and improved by exercise and gymnastic sports.

When, besides, people shall constantly breathe pure air, drink cold, pure water, eat simple, good food, wash and bathe, and keep themselves perfectly clean; and, by cultivation, render barren and unhealthful tracts of ground fertile and salubrious, and when Peace and Charity, guided by Reason and Virtue, shall extend their empire over the world—then, and then only, shall universal health and happiness prevail, and mankind enjoy the purest felicity.

But this glorious revolution in the manners, customs, and constitution of people of all descriptions, can hardly be expected to take place till that horrid pestilence called the small-pox is banished from the earth. That, then, it may soon be extirpated, and that this little book may increase universal felicity,

GRANT, ALMIGHTY GOD!

* *Dr. Benjamin Rush in Philadelphia confirms this truth.*

DECREE

DECREE

OF

HIS SERENE HIGHNESS

THE

PRINCE BISHOP OF WIRZBURGH,

TO THE

BAILIFFS OF THE HIGH METROPOLITAN CHURCH OF WIRZBURGH AND ITS DIOCESES,

CONCERNING

Dr. FAUST's
CATECHISM OF HEALTH.

His Serene Highness has ever considered the tenderest paternal care for the preservation of the health of his loyal subjects as his principal and noblest duty. In conformity to these principles he has employed every means of expelling from his bishopric all sorts of vagabonds and quacks, practising without any authority, and has actually established, even in the country, at certain proper distances, able physicians and surgeons.

However, as the appointing of such physicians and surgeons is not alone sufficient to make people who stand in need of medical assistance sensible of the necessity and utility of such regulations and instructions as tend to preserve and point out the mode of restoring health, it has been for a long time one of the most ardent wishes of His Serene Highness to see a doctrine of health introduced into schools and blended with the usual instructions.

His Highness by no means intends thereby to convert schoolmasters into doctors, or cause children to acquire any medical knowledge, but rather to make

K people

people attentive to their health; to instruct them how to esteem this great blessing, and how to preserve it; to acquaint them with the most usual maladies; to exterminate the very dangerous custom of self-treatment, and the making use of domestic remedies; and to make his subjects in general sensible of the indispensible necessity of committing themselves to the care of proper physicians and surgeons in all cases of illness.

The Catechism of Health of Dr. Faust, lately published, seemed to His Serene Highness the best book to answer these excellent purposes. He therefore was graciously pleased to order a very considerable number of copies (2000) to be bought and distributed gratis amongst the schoolmasters of his extensive dominions.

All bailiffs, therefore, are hereby strictly charged to transmit to each schoolmaster of every parish within their bailiwicks, one copy of the annexed Catechism of Health, with the following directions:

1. Each schoolmaster shall enter the copy sent to him in the common inventory of books, that it may be transferred to his successor.

2. Schoolmasters shall explain the different sections of the Catechism of Health once a week, at a certain time fixed by the curate or priest of the parish, and each time enter on a new subject.

3. Each section of the Catechism is to be transcribed by the children into their copy-books, that a more lasting impression may be made on their minds.

The bailiffs are particularly directed to remind schoolmasters of those directions; and His Highness positively orders that this business shall not only be strictly investigated at the monthly examinations, but also at the episcopal as well as school visitations. Decretum Wirzburgh, the 31st of December, 1793.

By Special Command of His Serene Highness,

To the Commissioners of Schools appointed by Episcopal Command.

INDEX.

INDEX.

	Page
ADDRESS to School-masters	3

FIRST DIVISION.
OF HEALTH.

I. Of Health; its Value, and the Duty of preserving it, and of instructing Mankind, particularly Children, in those important Subjects	7
II. Of the Duration of Life, and the Signs of Health	11
III. Of the Construction or Structure of the Human Body	13
IV. On the Attending and Nursing of Infants	16
V. Of the Treatment of Children with respect to their Bodies, from the Third to the Ninth or Twelfth Year	20
VI. Of Clothes fit to be worn by Children from the beginning of the Third to the End of the Seventh or Eighth Year; or till, in each of the two Jaws, the four weak Milk Teeth in Front are changed for four strong lasting Teeth	24
VII. Of Air	31
VIII. Of Cleanliness:—Washing and Bathing	33
IX. Of Food.	37
X. On Drink	43

XI. Of

	Page
XI. Of Wine	46
XII. Of Brandy	47
XIII. Of Tobacco	50
XIV. Of Exercise and Rest	ibid.
XV. Of Sleep	53
XVI. Of the Habitations of Man	56
XVII. Of Schools	58
XVIII. Of Thunder and Lightning	59
XIX. Of over-heating Ourselves, and catching Cold	60
XX. Of the Preservation of certain Parts of the Human Body	62
XXI. Of the Beauty and Perfection of the Human Body	66

SECOND DIVISION.
OF DISEASES.

XXII. Of Diseases; Physicians and Medicines	69
XXIII. Of the Conduct to be observed by Patients afflicted with Ardent Fevers	74
XXIV. Of Diseases which universally prevail; of Endemial, and of particular Maladies	83
XXV. Of Contagious Diseases	84
XXVI. Of the Small-pox	86
Instructions how to inoculate	88
XXVII. Of the Measles	90
XXVIII. On the entire Extirpation of the Small-pox and Measles	91
XXIX. Instructions how to exterminate the Small-pox by easy Means, in which every Individual is bound to concur	94
XXX. Of the Bloody Flux, or Dysentery	99
XXXI. Of Treatment, after Diseases are removed	100
XXXII. Of Public Institutions for the Sick	ibid.
Order of the Human Teeth	104
The Order and the Periods of Human Life	106
State of Perfect Health	108

FINIS

Medicine & Society In America

An Arno Press/New York Times Collection

Alcott, William A. **The Physiology of Marriage.** 1866. New Introduction by Charles E. Rosenberg.

Beard, George M. **American Nervousness: Its Causes and Consequences.** 1881. New Introduction by Charles E. Rosenberg.

Beard, George M. **Sexual Neurasthenia.** 5th edition. 1898.

Beecher, Catharine E. **Letters to the People on Health and Happiness.** 1855.

Blackwell, Elizabeth. **Essays in Medical Sociology.** 1902. Two volumes in one.

Blanton, Wyndham B. **Medicine in Virginia in the Seventeenth Century.** 1930.

Bowditch, Henry I. **Public Hygiene in America.** 1877.

Bowditch, N[athaniel] I. **A History of the Massachusetts General Hospital:** To August 5, 1851. 2nd edition. 1872.

Brill, A. A. **Psychanalysis:** Its Theories and Practical Application. 1913.

Cabot, Richard C. **Social Work:** Essays on the Meeting-Ground of Doctor and Social Worker. 1919.

Cathell, D. W. **The Physician Himself and What He Should Add to His Scientific Acquirements.** 2nd edition. 1882. New Introduction by Charles E. Rosenberg.

The Cholera Bulletin. Conducted by an Association of Physicians. Vol. I: Nos. 1–24. 1832. All published. New Introduction by Charles E. Rosenberg.

Clarke, Edward H. **Sex in Education;** or, A Fair Chance for the Girls. 1873.

Committee on the Costs of Medical Care. **Medical Care for the American People:** The Final Report of The Committee on the Costs of Medical Care, No. 28. [1932].

Currie, William. **An Historical Account of the Climates and Diseases of the United States of America.** 1792.

Davenport, Charles Benedict. **Heredity in Relation to Eugenics.** 1911. New Introduction by Charles E. Rosenberg.

Davis, Michael M. **Paying Your Sickness Bills.** 1931.

Disease and Society in Provincial Massachusetts: Collected Accounts, 1736–1939. 1972.

Earle, Pliny. **The Curability of Insanity:** A Series of Studies. 1887.

Falk, I. S., C. Rufus Rorem, and Martha D. Ring. **The Costs of Medical Care:** A Summary of Investigations on The Economic Aspects of the Prevention and Care of Illness, No. 27. 1933.

Faust, Bernhard C. **Catechism of Health:** For the Use of Schools, and for Domestic Instruction. 1794.

Flexner, Abraham. **Medical Education in the United States and Canada:** A Report to The Carnegie Foundation for the Advancement of Teaching, Bulletin Number Four. 1910.

Gross, Samuel D. **Autobiography of Samuel D. Gross, M.D.**, with Sketches of His Contemporaries. Two volumes. 1887.

Hooker, Worthington. **Physician and Patient;** or, A Practical View of the Mutual Duties, Relations and Interests of the Medical Profession and the Community. 1849.

Howe, S. G. **On the Causes of Idiocy.** 1858.

Jackson, James. **A Memoir of James Jackson, Jr., M.D.** 1835.

Jennings, Samuel K. **The Married Lady's Companion, or Poor Man's Friend.** 2nd edition. 1808.

The Maternal Physician; a Treatise on the Nurture and Management of Infants, from the Birth until Two Years Old. 2nd edition. 1818. New Introduction by Charles E. Rosenberg.

Mathews, Joseph McDowell. **How to Succeed in the Practice of Medicine.** 1905.

McCready, Benjamin W. **On the Influences of Trades, Professions, and Occupations in the United States, in the Production of Disease.** 1943.

Mitchell, S. Weir. **Doctor and Patient.** 1888.

Nichols, T[homas] L. **Esoteric Anthropology:** The Mysteries of Man. [1853].

Origins of Public Health in America: Selected Essays, 1820–1855. 1972.

Osler, Sir William. **The Evolution of Modern Medicine.** 1922.

The Physician and Child-Rearing: Two Guides, 1809–1894. 1972.

Rosen, George. **The Specialization of Medicine:** with Particular Reference to Ophthalmology. 1944.

Royce, Samuel. **Deterioration and Race Education.** 1878.

Rush, Benjamin. **Medical Inquiries and Observations.** Four volumes in two. 4th edition. 1815.

Shattuck, Lemuel, Nathaniel P. Banks, Jr., and Jehiel Abbott. **Report of a General Plan for the Promotion of Public and Personal Health.** Massachusetts Sanitary Commission. 1850.

Smith, Stephen. **Doctor in Medicine** and Other Papers on Professional Subjects. 1872.

Still, Andrew T. **Autobiography of Andrew T. Still,** with a History of the Discovery and Development of the Science of Osteopathy. 1897.

Storer, Horatio Robinson. **The Causation, Course, and Treatment of Reflex Insanity in Women.** 1871.

Sydenstricker, Edgar. **Health and Environment.** 1933.

Thomson, Samuel. **A Narrative, of the Life and Medical Discoveries of Samuel Thomson.** 1822.

Ticknor, Caleb. **The Philosophy of Living;** or, The Way to Enjoy Life and Its Comforts. 1836.

U.S. Sanitary Commission. **The Sanitary Commission of the United States Army:** A Succinct Narrative of Its Works and Purposes. 1864.

White, William A. **The Principles of Mental Hygiene.** 1917.